HEALING YOUR HEART

A Proven
Program for
Reversing
Heart Disease
Without
Drugs or
Surgery

HERMAN HELLERSTEIN, M.D.
AND PAUL PERRY

A Fireside Book,
Published by
SIMON & SCHUSTER   NEW YORK   LONDON   TORONTO   SYDNEY   TOKYO   SINGAPORE

FIRESIDE
Simon & Schuster Building
Rockefeller Center
1230 Avenue of the Americas
New York, New York 10020

First Fireside Edition 1991
FIRESIDE and colophon are registered trademarks of Simon &
Schuster Inc.

Designed by Barbara Marks Graphic Design
Manufactured in the United States of America

10   9   8   7   6   5   4   3   2   1
10   9   8   7   6   5   4   3   2   1   Pbk.

Library of Congress Cataloging in Publication Data
Hellerstein, Herman K.
    Healing your heart: a proven program for reversing heart disease
without drugs or surgery/Herman Hellerstein and Paul Perry.
        p.   cm.
    Includes bibliographical references.
    1. Coronary heart disease—Diet therapy.   2. Coronary heart
disease—Exercise therapy.   3. Coronary heart disease—Diet
therapy—Recipes.   I. Perry, Paul.   II. Title.
RC685.C6H43   1990
616.1′230654—dc20
DLC
for Library of Congress   90-9782
                                                                    CIP

ISBN 0-671-68323-3
ISBN 0-671-74802-5 Pbk.

To Mary F. Feil, M.D.
In memory of Mark C. McCourry
(1968–1989)

CONTENTS

TABLES

PART
I

PART
I

PART
I

CORONARY
HEART
DISEASE
CAN BE
REVERSED

*Seven Decades
of Research
Prove It*

1

In this age of health awareness, when so much attention is focused on the healthy heart, it is important to know that heart disease can be reversed. This is good news for us all, but especially for the seven out of ten American males over the age of thirty who have some signs of heart disease. And 40 percent of those with heart disease won't know it until they suddenly suffer a heart attack or death!

That coronary heart disease can be reversed has been known for more than seventy years, long before researchers even knew exactly why arteries became clogged or what they became clogged with. But over the past few years, with the improvement of techniques for measuring blood flow to the heart and the ability to examine X-ray photos of the heart, known as angiograms, it has become indisputable fact that much of the blockage that clogs the arteries is reversible, as well as modifiable and "stoppable."

In my forty-eight years as a cardiologist, I have seen reversal of heart disease many times. I have seen convincing evidence that the course of coronary disease which was previously thought to be relentless, could be slowed down, halted, and reversed. This has occurred in people who seemed destined for drastic treatment such as balloon angioplasty or a coronary bypass operation, as well as those who already had this remarkable surgery and did not relish another one.

I have seen and participated in the care of male and female patients where the course of coronary disease was literally reversed. The very concept of reversing coronary artery disease, of unblocking narrowed, plugged, or obstructed arteries sounds like an outrageous claim. The skeptics shout, "Can you unfry an egg?" "Can you reverse time?" The answer to both of these questions is a qualified "yes." Let me give you an example of how this works in another type of heart disease, a tremendous enlargement of the heart muscle called cardiac hypertrophy. This is due to the increased work of the heart that occurs in people with high blood pressure or narrowed heart valves. Reduction of the heart workload can result in gradual return of the heart to normal, and the heart muscle cells can decrease in size. The electro-cardiogram, the chest X-ray shadows, and heart functions often revert to completely normal, as though the heart had never been enlarged. Time cannot be reversed, but the physical decline that we associate with aging can be reversed. Physiologic time can be and often is reversible.

The reversal of coronary artery disease can be accomplished with a program of proper nutrition, exercise, no smoking, and stress (really strain) reduction that is no more restrictive or more strenuous than most enlightened cardiologists now recommend. Many of you may be living a preventive or partial-reversal life-style now. Many of you may have to make only small and prudent changes in your life-style. Some of you may have to make substantially larger changes, but they are changes well worth the effort, since decades of medical research have substantiated without doubt that one can undo much of the clogging ravages of atherosclerosis. In the process, you will lose weight, or at least you will lose excessive body fat if you need to. You will look better and feel healthier and more energetic.

In my own research at the Case Western Reserve University, involving almost 1,000 patients with heart disease, I have seen heart disease reversed. All of the patients who started in two major research projects were afflicted with serious and documented coronary heart disease. Yet, in a matter of only six weeks on the program, the majority of them showed significant signs of improvement. At the end of the three-year study of the multicenter federally funded National Exercise and Heart Disease project we had scientific proof that the circulatory system grew physiologically "younger," reversing the deteriorating effects of age and heart disease. Similar observations were found in the earlier Cleveland Jewish Community—Case Western Reserve University project.

This book presents the reversal diet program and explains how to fit it into your life-style. In fact, the word "diet" means more than just what you eat. It means your daily "regimen" or system of eating, as well as your exercises and responses to the stresses of living.

I will outline the seven goals for reversal and show briefly how each can contribute to the reversal of heart disease. Following that I will show you how to examine your own life-style to see how close you now are to the program we recommend.

The remainder of the book offers in-depth advice on meeting the seven reversal goals:

- A total serum cholesterol of 200 mg/dl or less, with a total cholesterol to HDL cholesterol ratio of 3.5 to 1 or less with LDL cholesterol less than 130 mg/dl
- Normal blood pressure
- Regular exercise (and I will define what this means)
- Body weight within 5 percent of normal
- Coping with stress without strainful response
- No tobacco—period!
- Normal blood-sugar levels

But before we look at how each of these factors can work miracles in your body, let's look at the history of reversal research.

What Builds Up, Can Build Down

In 1961, the American Heart Association took a bold position in the war against coronary heart disease. In a report entitled, "Dietary Fat and Its Relation to Heart Attacks and Strokes," it concluded that saturated fat, the type found mainly in animal products, causes a rise in blood cholesterol that results in an increased rate of atherosclerotic coronary heart disease.

"When the intake of saturated fats is reduced, blood cholesterol levels usually decrease," read the report. "When [unsaturated] fats are substituted for a substantial part of the saturated fats . . . blood cholesterol decreases."

This official report—the first of its kind to come from the AHA—was based on decades of suspicion by medical science that animal fat was the chief cause of heart disease. Researchers knew that when these saturated fats were easily accessible, the number of people suffering from heart disease rose substantially. And they knew that when animal fats were restricted, fewer people had heart disease.

But what was most interesting to many was another of their findings: heart disease could be reversed! Given significant reductions in blood cholesterol and adequate time, the blockages that choke the life out of the heart could actually be reduced in size. This was particularly exciting news. Rather than thinking of heart disease as a progressive malady that only became worse, medical science and the general public could look at it as a dynamic process, one for which there could be hope for improvement.

This exciting notion was not new, even in 1961. It had been presented many times. The notion that heart disease was reversible was first put forth by S. W. Aschoff in 1924. This research physician examined postmortem reports from World War I and concluded that atherosclerotic lesions—the blockages that form in arteries—might be reversed by the type of low-fat diet followed during the war years.

In 1932, Dr. Wilhelm Raab drew the same conclusion as Aschoff did. He showed that atherosclerosis and heart disease dropped during World War I in the populations where eggs, milk, butter, and meat became less available. He compared these findings to the few studies linking animal fats to heart disease and concluded that these saturated fats were the culprits that clogged veins and arteries. Take them away and life-threatening blockages stop growing and sometimes almost disappear, he concluded.

Too much animal fat could cause heart disease. That was quite a revelation for a country that revered its bacon and eggs, at a time when most people regarded a diet high in animal fat to be as harmless as cigarettes, which, as the advertisements of the day declared, "warmed your lungs" and were good for colds and emphysema. Too much animal fat as a heart-stopper? Let the researchers eat cake if they didn't like good old American farm products.

A Farewell to Heart Disease

With World War II research into the reversibility of heart disease continued. But there were few volunteers for this experimentation, just forced participants.

The protocol for many of the "experiments" went as follows: the German army took over a country and immediately seized control of the food supplies from the countryside. They would keep the meat, eggs, milk, and cheese for themselves. Limited amounts of the rest of the food—wheat, vegetables, and the like—were given to the locals.

The Germans conducted this military "experiment" in Belgium, Holland, Poland, and Norway. These enforced dietary changes caused some obvious outward changes in the people who lived in these countries. They lost body weight. Many became physiologically stronger by virtue of having less fat to lug around. Cars were usually confiscated or forced to become idle without gasoline supplies, and the people had to walk or ride bicycles everywhere. Surprisingly, many who were fed on the "lesser" foods that the Germans allowed them found that they functioned better on this "poor" diet. They lost weight and had a sense of being stronger.

But these dietary changes caused some unseen changes in the populations of these countries, too. In country after country where eating habits were changed by the German military occupation, the rate of heart disease plummeted. Where autopsies were performed, dramatic reversal of atherosclerotic lesions were shown. This didn't mean that war was good for the heart, but it did mean that the wartime diet was, despite the terror of occupation and the undernutrition.

For instance, in Rotterdam's municipal hospitals in 1945, coronary deaths were one-fifth those of the prewar years. This led researcher Dr. H. E. Schornagle to conclude, "the decrease in coronary [death] is closely related to the nutritional intake . . . particularly to a diet which has been rich in fat." This reduction in heart disease resulted *despite* the emotional stress of occupation.

In Norway, the number of heart-disease patients in Porsgrunn's Hospital before the war was 3 percent of total admissions. During the war these admissions dropped to half that percentage.

In Finland, Dr. I. Vartianen compared heart-attack rates from 1936 through the war years and concluded that the least amount of heart disease occurred in 1944 when fatty foods were most restricted.

In Russia, where the Germans captured much of the food, a "marked reduction was found in the incidence of angina pectoris and coronary occlusion" during the blockade of Leningrad in 1941–42. Dr. K. G. Volkova, reporting these findings in Moscow's *Clinical Medicine,* attributed the lower rate to a reduction in dietary fat.

The Germans found themselves the subjects of some dietary "experimentation," too, at the hands of the Russians. Germans captured on the Russian front were treated harshly by their captors, taken to prison camps, and fed a starvation diet.

Dr. George Schettler, a German cardiologist and prison doctor in one of these Russian POW camps, was allowed to perform autopsies on his countrymen who died while imprisoned. "On hundreds of autopsies, there was very little evidence of any atherosclerosis," he told a symposium at the New York Academy of Sciences in 1961.

"[The disappearance of lesions] was due to the effects of the low-fat diet given the German prisoners by the Russians."

Dr. Schettler added: "In Germany in the final years of World War II, I was told by my colleagues that it was difficult to obtain examples of individuals with atherosclerosis for demonstration to the medical students."

Blockages Make a Comeback

Finding blocked arteries became easier after the war. When the saturated fat of eggs, butter, milk, and red meat found its way back to these "nutritionally deprived" nations, the disease of prosperity found its way back to their hearts.

I personally witnessed this phenomenon in some of the survivors of the Bergen-Belsen concentration camp as a member of the U.S. Seventh Armored Division. Although most had lost all the symptoms of their heart disease while prisoners, many were heavy and sick when I had an opportunity to reexamine them ten years later. Coronary artery disease had returned; they had eaten their way back to illness.

Dr. William Castelli, director of the Framingham Heart Study in Massachusetts, often recalls his postwar experience in a Belgium hospital. Before the war, atherosclerotic lesions were present in 60 to 70 percent of all autopsies they conducted. Yet by 1942 these lesions had almost entirely disappeared. "They couldn't even show a pathology resident what the most common pathological lesion looked like," Castelli remarked.

Yet in the 1950s while working for a pathologist in Belgium, Castelli saw heart disease return. While the two of them performed autopsies, the pathologist would frequently shake his head and say, "It's coming back."

"What's coming back?" asked Castelli.

"The atherosclerosis," said the pathologist.

The disease had largely disappeared between 1942 and around 1950. But now it was returning to its prewar levels.

It became easier to find arterial blockage in other countries, too. Dr. Fritz Pezold examined 6,000 autopsy reports in Berlin. He found severe coronary blockage in five out of ten autopsies when the wartime German diet averaged 8 percent fat. But in the early fifties, when the average consumption of fat was up to 30 percent of the calories (much of it saturated fat), severe blockage was found in eight out of ten autopsies.

Dr. Schettler, the prison-camp doctor, witnessed an increase in heart disease, too. He found that "dozens of cases" of heart disease developed in the soldiers he had treated in Russia. He knew this because he continued to treat them after the war. Gradually, over the decade after the war, these formerly starved POWs came back to Schettler suffering from their regained prosperity. "They went back to their high-fat diet," he said. "And dozens of cases of coronary disease developed."

From Porsgrunn, Norway, and Rotterdam, Holland, the results were the same: atherosclerosis had returned. In Japan, the rate of heart attacks has climbed dramatically since World War II. This rise in coronary artery disease is strongly linked to the adoption of the Western diet.

These nutritional experiments conducted through the nightmare of war gave credence to Dr. Wilhelm Raab's 1932 assertion: saturated fat clogs the arteries. Decrease saturated fat in your diet and you literally reverse your chances of heart disease.

But these nutritional changes also showed significant proof of Aschoff's notion from 1924: atherosclerosis—the actual blockage in the arteries—could be reversed by following a diet low in saturated fat.

Research interest was piqued. Many questions about the reversibility of heart disease came to the fore:

- **What level of blood cholesterol was required to achieve reversal?**
- **Did a "reversal" diet always stop or at least reduce the chance of heart disease?**
- **What effect does exercise have on artery blockage? Does it reverse damage already done by heart disease or hurt the damaged heart muscle even more?**

Researching Reversal

In the decades since the war, reversal research has increased many-fold. Using a variety of medical tools and testing a number of hypotheses about the buildup of blockage and how it can be reversed, medical scientists have been learning new ways of fighting back against America's number-one killer, heart disease.

As with all good medical research, progress is slow because it must be meticulous. Yet after hundreds of experiments conducted on thousands of human and animal subjects I can say with assurance that coronary heart disease is reversible. The medical literature proves it, and I have seen it happen in many of my own patients. These decades of research have shown that:

• *Atherosclerosis is a dynamic process.* As blockages build up, so can they reduce in size. In some ways you can compare these changes to changes in your waistline (although the two aren't necessarily related since thin people also experience heart disease albeit less frequently). Your waistline grows and shrinks, depending upon the type and amount of food you eat. The same is often true of blockages in arteries. Granted, some blockages "calcify," especially older ones. But even these contain reversible components like fat deposits and blood clots.

• *Simple changes in diet and exercise may accomplish reversal.* It is often not necessary to go on a severely restricted diet or a strict exercise regimen to reduce cholesterol levels. I have found with my patients that changes in just a few habits are often all that is necessary to reduce harmful blood-cholesterol levels substantially. For instance, some people can just reduce the amount of fast foods they eat—or the type—and lower cholesterol levels. Others can replace eggs with egg substitutes and reduce their cholesterol count. Most people, I have found, eat well, with only minor exceptions to an otherwise healthy diet. The vigorous public education programs of the American Heart Association and National Heart Institute are proving successful, as shown by the more than 25 percent *decrease* in the death rate from coronary artery disease between the years of 1955 and 1985.

• *Physiological aging can be reversed.* Although it is impossible to reverse chronological aging (the actual passing of time), it is possible to reverse the functional aspects of physiological aging. For instance,

I have sixty-year-old heart patients who are in better shape than the average forty year old. Again, they have accomplished this physical feat with few changes, and usually pleasant ones at that. By following their exercise prescription, they experience the vitality that activity gives them. Not only are they feeling better, but they are also functioning better on the treadmill tests. They *feel* twenty years younger because they are *functioning* as if they were years younger.

How Atherosclerosis Builds

Most patients are surprised by the improvements in their arteries when they make the changes I recommend. They conceive of heart disease as something that always becomes progressively worse. The mention of clogged arteries to patients conjures up some obvious images. Some think that fat and cholesterol accumulate in arteries like cooking fat that is allowed to congeal in the pipes of a kitchen sink. Others think of atherosclerosis as being like a hairball that clogs the bath drain and keeps water from draining out.

But atherosclerosis is quite different from the clogging of pipes. It usually occurs slowly over the course of several years, even decades. Sometimes it regresses on its own and other times it builds faster than would be expected. But the factors that control the clogging of arteries are always present long before the symptoms of the disease. They work silently until blood flow becomes so restricted that chest pain or a heart attack announces the unwelcome presence of heart disease.

The buildup that chokes arteries is composed of cholesterol, fat, fibrous tissue, smooth muscle, clotted blood, and calcium. And although it can eventually restrict the flow of blood, it starts not in the blood vessel where the blood flows but in the walls of the vessels themselves.

It is when the delicate lining of the artery walls is irritated by such things as cholesterol and saturated fats or the cracking pressure of hypertension that the atherosclerotic process begins. When these irritants are removed, atherosclerosis starts to disappear. How much of it disappears depends upon the amount and type of blockage that is present. Artery blockages don't occur in a uniform fashion like the layers of a cake. Instead they happen in patches, plaques, and layers. The speed with which atherosclerosis can reverse depends upon its age, composition, and the factors that are working to eliminate it. "New" atherosclerosis is usually made of fat and cholesterol and is much easier to reverse than an "old" one that includes calcium and connective tissue. But all begin essentially the same way.

INTIMAL IRRITATION

Arteries have three layers: the outside layer is the adventitia, a tough layer of connective tissue that covers the artery like the insulation on an electrical wire. The next layer, the media, is smooth muscle that constricts or dilates, depending upon its stimulus. For instance, anger can cause arteries to constrict and raise blood pressure. Relaxation allows them to dilate or open up, reducing blood pressure.

The layer on the inside of the artery is the endothelium. This layer consists of intima cells that look square and uniform resembling tiles on a floor when viewed through a microscope.

It is in the intimal layer that atherosclerosis begins. Intima is smooth like glass. But when these tiny "tiles" are disrupted, the buildup begins.

The cause of disruption is a type of cholesterol known as low density lipoprotein (LDL). It consists of *large* globules of cholesterol encapsulated in a thin protein shell. *Small* globules of cholesterol, high density lipoprotein (HDL), are credited with attaching themselves to LDLs and pulling them into the bloodstream and transporting them out of the body. But when there are more LDLs than the HDLs can manage, the intima becomes damaged. For reasons that aren't totally understood, the LDLs lodge in the intima. There they begin to accumulate in the cracked and broken "tile."

The accumulation of cholesterol underneath the intima was actually witnessed by Dr. C. M. W. Adams at the Guys Hospital Medical School in London in 1962. At that time there were still some skeptical scientists who didn't believe that blood cholesterol was responsible for atherosclerosis. They theorized that artery walls chemically manufactured the cholesterol found in the blockages and that it didn't come from the blood at all.

To test both hypotheses, Adams fed radioactive cholesterol to animals. He was then able to document with sophisticated equipment as the "tagged" cholesterol moved from the blood to the intimal lining. This experiment gave photographic proof that the cholesterol in atherosclerosis came from the blood. It also showed the damage that cholesterol does to the intima.

These fatty "streaks" have been shown to start early in life, in the teens or earlier especially in our meat-eating, deep-fried society. Autopsies performed on 300 young American soldiers killed in the Korean War revealed that 77 percent had some atherosclerosis. In contrast, Korean soldiers killed in the same battle had one-tenth as many lesions. This high rate of blockage was attributed to a military and civilian diet rich in saturated fats.

SWOLLEN WITH CONNECTIVE TISSUE

This disruption in blood flow and the surface smoothness of the intima inspire other elements of atherosclerosis. Smooth-muscle cells begin to form around and behind the still-growing cholesterol deposits, pushing the atheroma into the lumen, or vessel itself, where it starts to interfere with blood flow. Calcium may also form in the atheroma at this point, possibly because of its electrical attraction to cholesterol.

As the artery becomes narrower, blood flows faster and with more velocity through the restricted area. Adrenaline in the bloodstream makes the surface of the atheroma rough like ground glass. This body-produced chemical does wonders to speed the heart rate and raise blood pressure when we are excited or angry, but on a growing atheroma it acts like sandpaper to make the surface coarse.

The change in the atheroma's surface starts a whole new phase of buildup—blood clotting.

The building block of the blood clot is a dumbbell-shaped molecule called fibrinogen. When blood is leaked from the circulatory system, whether it be from a bloody nose or a gunshot wound, fibrinogen appears and links together with blood elements to form fibrin, which acts as a sort of bridge over the wound.

As the fibrin bridge is formed, blood platelets are attracted from the blood to the edges of the blood-vessel wall. These disc-shaped cells increase in number with fibrinogen until a clot has formed that can plug the hemorrhage while healing takes place.

Why a clot forms on the rough surface of an atheroma isn't fully

understood. But it is known that the level of fibrinogen is higher in patients with signs of heart disease than in those who are free of such signs. It is also known that blood in a test tube with a roughened spot on its inner surface will form a clot on that spot. This is why atheromas are often topped with a blood clot that block an artery and start the catastrophe known as a heart attack. When this occurs in an artery in the brain a stroke occurs.

"Seeing" Reversal

As far as I know, the first scientist to see reversal in action was Dr. David Rutstein in the 1950s. This Harvard University researcher wanted to see just how blockage actually grew in a test tube. At the time he was studying steroids and their effects upon "living" specimens of artery walls that he was growing in test-tube cultures. Because cholesterol is chemically related to this class of drugs, Rutstein used it as part of the test.

To Rutstein's great surprise the cholesterol seemed to be entering the cell walls when it was tested on the artery tissue.

Rutstein was intrigued. He launched a series of tests in which everything suspected of causing artery blockage was tested. He tested cholesterol, lipoproteins, and saturated and unsaturated fats. He watched through an electron microscope as cholesterol entered the smooth intimal cells that line the artery. When a solution high in cholesterol and saturated fat was used, the cholesterol was deposited at a faster rate. When cholesterol and unsaturated fats were mixed and placed in test tubes with the arteries, the unsaturated fats prevented the growth of lesions.

Then Rutstein did something fascinating. He took a piece of the living artery tissue that had the beginning of atherosclerosis and put it into a bath of blood with a low-cholesterol count. *The cholesterol left the intima,* an example of reverse transport. In a test tube, he watched atherosclerosis reverse.

Since then there have been many experiments showing that the blockages of the heart can be reversed. They almost all come to the same conclusion: under certain conditions, atherosclerotic plaque (or deposits) is a reversible lesion.

Direct Observation on Animals

From the 1920s to the present, the reversal of atherosclerotic lesions has been witnessed many times in animals.

Although S. W. Aschoff in 1924 may have been the first physician to conclude that atherosclerosis is reversible, N. N. Antischkow was probably the first to show it. In the 1940s, he fed rabbits a high-cholesterol diet and then sacrificed some of them to examine their arteries surgically. He found well-developed coronary lesions. He then changed the diet of the remaining rabbits, feeding them the low-cholesterol fare that rabbits usually eat. After several weeks he sacrificed the remaining rabbits and examined their arteries. In them he found lesions that were smaller in size and fat content than those of the previously examined rabbits.

This type of experiment has been repeated many times in numerous animals, including chickens, dogs, pigeons, pigs, and monkeys.

For example, in one study pigs were fed a high-cholesterol diet for four months. Some of them were then sacrificed to determine how much cholesterol-containing plaque had built up in their aortas.

The remaining pigs were then fed a diet for fourteen months that was free of cholesterol. At the end of that period they were autopsied. Although some buildup remained, it was considerably less than that found in the first group. The researchers also noted that the remaining plaques had caused less arterial damage than the blockages in the first group that had not been given a chance to reverse.

Here at Case Western Reserve University, an even more direct demonstration of reversal was carried out in 1970 by Dr. Ralph De-Palma, who is now a professor of surgery at George Washington University. He and his associate Dr. William Insull fed high-cholesterol diets to dogs for a period of several weeks. The atherosclerotic lesions produced from this diet were surgically exposed, stained, and photographed. The arteries were then surgically repaired to restore blood flow.

DePalma then fed one group of dogs a low-fat, low-cholesterol diet to defat them. He continued to feed the other group the lesion-producing diet. After several more weeks, both groups were sacrificed and their atherosclerotic lesions examined and photographed. The dogs that had been defatted showed a substantial reduction in the size of their lesions. The dogs fed the high-cholesterol, high-fat diet had lesions that grew worse.

HAVE YOUR CAKE AND EAT IT, TOO

In the past decade, M. René Malinow, a researcher at the Oregon Primate Research Center, has begun experimenting with something known as a bile sequestrant. This remarkable substance keeps cholesterol from entering the bloodstream by binding with it in the stomach and intestines. It then holds on to pass the cholesterol out of the body. Bile sequestrants can be taken medicinally in a pure form, but they are also found naturally in such foods as oatmeal, bran, and fruits and vegetables. When eaten in smaller amounts in foods such as oat-bran muffins or cereal, bile sequestrants can be considered food. When taken in concentrated form on a regular basis, bile sequestrants can be considered medicine.

Malinow wondered: what would happen if one were fed a high-cholesterol diet that was mixed with a bile sequestrant? To answer this question, Malinow has conducted several primate experiments, feeding monkeys a high-cholesterol diet mixed with alfalfa meal, an excellent bile sequestrant. All of his studies have shown a remarkable decrease in the size of lesions in monkeys when bile sequestrants are used.

What this means is that simple changes in diet—the eating of more bran or cereals instead of saturated fats, for instance, or the daily drinking of a bile sequestrant mixed in a glass of orange juice—can reduce cholesterol and the amount of blockage in the arteries. This isn't all you need to do to reverse heart disease most effectively. But it does show that just reducing blood cholesterol can reduce the size of lesions and your chances of new ones.

SPACE-AGE VIEW

With the development and improvement of imaging equipment, the inside of the human body can now be viewed without surgery or other invasive techniques. Improvements in angiography, the procedure that allows us to examine arteries with dyes and X rays, have permitted researchers to see changes in human lesions as they occur.

One such study using improved angiography was done by Dr. David Blankenhorn at the University of Southern California. He was actually able to capture on film the regression of lesions in nine patients placed on cholesterol-lowering drugs.

In a landmark study conducted by Dr. Henry Buchwald of the University of Minnesota School of Medicine, twenty-two hypercholesterolemic patients (people whose bodies produce dangerously high amounts of cholesterol) were given intestinal bypass surgery to keep cholesterol out of their systems. A series of arteriograms for three years after surgery showed that 14 percent of the patients had regression of their coronary atherosclerosis while 55 percent showed no change. The reversed lesions speak for themselves. But merely stopping the growth of lesions, especially in people with serious hypercholesterolemia, is reversal in itself.

Another study to examine the effects of lowered serum cholesterol on atherosclerosis was conducted by the National Heart, Lung and Blood Institute. Patients with very high cholesterol levels and signs of coronary artery disease were placed on low-fat, low-cholesterol diets. Half of the patients were then selected to receive six grams, four times a day, of a bile-sequestrant drug. The other half received a placebo, which is a substance that has no medicinal or nutritional value. They were all then given coronary arteriograms.

Several years later the arteriograms were repeated. The group that received the bile sequestrant had significantly less progression of disease. And most important, among those with lesions that blocked the arteries by 50 percent or greater, only 12 percent of the patients treated with bile sequestrants got worse. In the group that didn't lower its serum-cholesterol levels, almost three times as many worsened.

An equally impressive prospective randomized study, by skeptical investigators who doubted that coronary artery disease was reversible, was conducted by Dr. B. Greg Brown and associates at the University of Washington, Seattle. They provided unequivocal evidence of significant regression of coronary atherosclerosis and of cardiac events in 66 men over a period of 2.5 years, compared to a control group of 37 men with conventional therapy. These favorable changes in the clinical course and severity of coronary lesions were brought about by decreases in LDL cholesterol and increases in HDL cholesterol, produced by a combination of diet, bile sequestrant, and either lovastatin (Mevacor) or Colestipol (Colestid).

Another pioneering study that has made great use of space-age imaging technology is currently being conducted by investigators in San Francisco and in Houston. Entitled "Adherence and Lifestyle Changes and Reversal of Coronary Atherosclerosis" and headed by Dr. Dean Ornish, an internist at the UCSF Medical School, its purpose was to examine the effects of very drastic life-style changes on patients with coronary artery disease.

The participants in Ornish's San Francisco study were independently evaluated by Dr. K. Lance Gould and associates in Houston. The control group received the usual care and advice about reducing dietary cholesterol and no smoking. The experimental group received *no medication,* but was provided and expected to adhere to a vegetarian diet that was very low in saturated fat (10 percent fat calories) and unusually low in cholesterol (5 mg), to exercise moderately three times a week, and to participate in stress-management techniques like yoga, meditation, and group counseling several times a week—total involvement of more than 15 hours per week.

At the November 1989 American Heart Association meeting, Ornish reported that 29 patients with 142 coronary lesions had gone through one yearlong program and had completed quantitative coronary angiography at baseline and after one year. Their cholesterol counts had dropped from an average of 237 to 136 mg/dl. The experimental group showed regression (about 4 percent less narrowing of the average diameter of the coronary lesions). Meanwhile the control group had worsened, showing an average increase of 2 percent of average diameter narrowing.

Gould, Ornish, and associates also reported on 57 patients with 269 coronary artery narrowings (stenosis) who were studied before and after a one- to two-year period, as a control or on lipid (fat)-lowering protocol. Significant regression and improvement in coronary blood flow and heart-muscle perfusion occurred in the subjects with total cholesterol less than 200 mg/dl and LDL cholesterol less than 130 mg/dl. In contrast significant progression of blockages occurred when total cholesterol was more than 200 mg/dl and the LDL cholesterol was more than 130 mg/dl.

But perhaps even more impressive recent research by Dr. Blankenhorn at USC demonstrated the positive beneficial effects of life-style changes far less stringent and demanding, compared to the complexity and time commitment of those in Ornish's investigation. In the past Blankenhorn has successfully reversed heart disease by having patients use cholesterol-lowering drugs and make life-style changes. But at the 1988 meeting of the American Heart Association he reported a non-drug study in which eighty-two patients were given extensive nutritional counseling and advised to reduce their daily fat intake to about 27 percent of their total calories.

As Dr. Blankenhorn told the *Washington Post* later: "We find that the ones who reduced their total fat intake, their saturated fat intake, and their cholesterol intake did not form new coronary lesions.

"These guys were not starving. They did not lose weight. They were selecting what they wanted to eat. The important change that they made was the reduction of high-fat foods."

This very careful researcher went on to make a very important statement: "To just stop [or reverse] the formation of lesions that block vessels to the heart, you may not have to make big changes in your diet."

THE REVERSAL PROGRAM: MY OWN RESEARCH

What does all of this painstaking research mean? It means that the progression of heart disease isn't inevitable. It means that you have considerable control over your heart's health. It means that with knowledge and some self-care you can slow down, halt, and even reverse the atherosclerotic process.

I told you in the beginning of this chapter that I have seen this reversed many times in my own patients. Now let me tell you about my own involvement with the regression of heart disease.

After the war I studied with famed pathologists Howard Karsner and Harry Goldblatt at the Institute of Pathology at Cleveland's Case Western Reserve University. There I was able to witness firsthand the regression of heart disease in civilians similar to those in concentration camps.

In one such study I examined the hearts from 2,000 consecutive autopsies to determine how often various diseases of the heart occur. I found cardiac lesions to be present in almost half of the patients autopsied. Significant coronary disease was found in 23 percent of the autopsy population. Although all of these lesions didn't necessarily contribute to death, 19 percent of the total autopsy population and 39 percent of the cases with heart disease died directly from heart failure.

I discovered something else, too. The arteries of those people who had died of "wasting diseases" like cancer and anorexia nervosa were defatted and relatively clear of atherosclerotic lesions in the coronary arteries and aorta. Some scar tissue remained, especially in those hearts that we traced back to people with a history of serious heart problems before the onset of their wasting disease. But for the most part, coronary-artery blockages had decreased.

I made another amazing discovery: the muscle fibers in the hearts of those people with high blood pressure before their final illness were back to normal size. Hypertension—high blood pressure—leads to enlarged muscle fibers, a condition known as hypertrophy. But when the people I studied lost weight, their blood pressure decreased and many of those fibers in their hearts were no longer enlarged. In the few that were enlarged, the change for the better was remarkable.

I speculated in the published report in 1950 that: "Hence it is conceivable that there are clinical conditions in which it would be desirable to accomplish this [reversal of heart disease] by controlled *undernutrition* [not malnutrition] to decrease cardiac work.

"The permanency of these gains and the problems of rehabilitation should be determined by clinical trials."

The recovery by refeeding of experimentally starved animals and humans and of inmates of concentration camps indicate the reversibility of atrophy of the heart and body, from atrophy toward normal.

Thus, both hypertrophy and atrophy of the heart are reversible.

After leaving the CWRU Institute of Pathology, I witnessed, as a research fellow, impressive reversibility of atherosclerosis produced by animal experiments at the famous laboratory of Louis N. Katz at the Michael Reese Cardiovascular Institute in Chicago.

Some researchers fed chickens a diet that was high in cholesterol. Within eight months the chickens developed heart-choking lesions. When these chickens were surgically examined, they had blockages that were as bad or worse than those of an eighty-year-old man.

The researchers then reversed the atherosclerosis in the chickens by putting them on low-cholesterol diets and giving them estrogen, the hormone that protects most women from heart disease.

I now knew why chickens don't eat eggs; they just laid them and walked away. I also knew for certain what many other researchers already knew, that atherosclerosis could be reversed.

From Observation to Intervention

In 1950 I established a multidisciplinary Work Classification Clinic to evaluate heart patients, their cardiovascular function, their emotional and psychological adjustments, and to advise them in regards to returning to work. In a thirteen-year period, over 90 percent of 2,000 patients were able to return to gainful employment, in a great variety of jobs—successfully, safely, and without work-related litigation. I learned through systematic followup that the patients who returned to vigorous recreational and occupational work became more fit, less overweight, less depressed and survived better than patients with the same severity of heart disease who maintained a more restricted life-style, although advised otherwise!

The fifties and sixties were the epidemic years for heart disease. These days we can expect to lose 514,000 people a year to heart disease alone, not counting 149,000 strokes, 31,000 due to high blood pressure. Had the high rates of twenty and thirty years ago continued, we would now be losing an estimated 870,000 people per year.

Because of this epidemic of heart disease, I helped conceive and codirect a multicenter study for the U.S. Department of Health, Education Administration called the National Exercise and Heart Disease Project. In part, the NEHDP came out of a smaller study I had conducted in the 1960s in Cleveland that examined the effects of exercise and life-style change on a sample of 654 men who had already had heart disease or were prone to getting it. We studied men because 90–95 percent of heart attacks before the age of fifty occur in men. We weren't discriminating against women; nature was already discriminating on their behalf.

In the study we had 254 patients who had already been stricken with heart disease and nearly 400 who were coronary prone.

I assembled a team of physicians, psychologists, psychiatrists, anthropologists, dieticians, exercise physiologists, and nurses who could examine virtually every aspect of the participants' lives.

We gave the patients personality tests to establish the type of people they were and to see if they were depressed or anxious or needed special help in order to participate in a life-style–change program.

We had the participants keep detailed food diaries for at least a week so the dietician could analyze the content of their diets. That way we could tell them what to change (if anything) and possibly help them alter their fat and cholesterol levels without greatly changing the composition of their meals.

We also did somatyping, which photographically determines the type of body shape a person has. This was important in following their body shapes as they lost weight and also in deciding which type of exercise they should do. For instance, people with big bellies and little legs shouldn't be running intensely; they should take advantage of their flotation by swimming. For them, running might cause joint injury.

We then prescribed exercise with the same precision with which we prescribe medicine. What we were looking for was a minimum effective dose. Too little wouldn't have much effect on metabolism or oxygen uptake. But too much might be harmful or unacceptable to the patients with heart disease. They were expected to show up three times a week at the program's workout center to do at least thirty minutes of exercise per session under direct supervision.

The patients came from all walks of life, and all were treated equally. We established a "buddy" system for the exercise program. It wasn't uncommon for a porter to call the president of a company, for instance, and ask him why he'd missed that day's exercise session. Because of this strong buddy system and supervision, the exercise classes had a retention rate of almost 90 percent, whereas about 60 percent of the participants usually drop out of most classes of that kind.

After only three years of participation, the results were astonishing. The mortality rate was reduced, the number of heart attacks was reduced and survival was enhanced.

In the National Exercise and Heart Disease Project, the mortality rate was 36.5 percent lower in the exercise group than in the control nonexercise group. Similar benefits were later reported by Roy Shephard, who combined the results of three prospective randomized controlled studies of the effects of exercise on cardiac patients in the United States, Sweden, and Finland. They showed comparable reduction in mortality and morbidity. We accomplished these beneficial effects by reducing the subjects' body weight to within 5 to 8 percent of normal percent body fat, reducing the total cholesterol and elevation of HDL cholesterol in the blood, and we used exercise to increase their bodies' capacity to work, that is, aerobic capacity, thus making them physiologically younger than their chronologic age.

On the whole, it was easy for these patients to achieve a longer and healthier life. In an eight-year followup of the Case Western Reserve University participating subjects, the mortality rate was less than two per hundred participants per year, which implies that the average participant can expect to survive at least twenty-five years after the heart attack that entered him into the study. All that was required were simple life-style changes.

LIVING PROOF OF REVERSAL

Let me offer some "before and after" examples of a few people who participated in this program.

One patient—we'll call him James—was forty-two when he had those sharp pains in his chest known as angina pectoris. This was his first sign of heart disease, but it wasn't the first time it had appeared in his family. Every male member of his family had died of heart disease before the age of forty-five. With a family history like that, his chances of living past fifty were slim indeed.

Patients sometimes become angry when physicians tell them that the odds in life are very much against them. But James was reasonable. Rather than display anger, he wanted to know what I could do—if anything—to push the odds more in his favor.

I told him what I could do. "We'll exercise you, defat you, and desmoke you. And we'll help you gain a better insight into what you can do to keep your heart healthy."

That was more than twenty years ago. Over the years he has developed into a fine athlete by doing everything in his power to reverse the trend of heart-disease death in his family. His wife has helped him, too, encouraging him to exercise and eat right. He has far outlived his expected life span as predicted by his family history. He outlived his father's age of death and that of his brother, who always thought it was nonsense that heart disease could be reversed.

Another of my patients—we'll call him Tom—wasn't so pleasant when he was told that the odds were two out of three that he would have a heart attack in the next five years.

The reasons were as clear as the data that prediction was based upon. Tom was forty years old and weighed 280 pounds. According to the height/weight charts, he was at least 100 pounds overweight (or 12 inches too short). He couldn't walk more than a few yards without becoming short of breath. He was a chain smoker. As far as his heart went, Tom had little going for him.

He was angry when I pointed out the odds against him. He thought I was being negative and judgmental and left my office declaring that there was nothing wrong with the way he lived his life. A few days later he came back and joined the program.

After two years of adherence to the program, Tom beat the odds. He lost 110 pounds, stopped smoking, and found great joy in regular exercise. Best of all, time has shown that he has clearly beaten the five-year prediction of a heart attack.

Immunize Now Against Heart Disease

There are hundreds of stories like these from my programs and among my patients, people who reversed their heart disease and are living today because of these simple yet effective life-style changes.

None of these success stories surprises me. Seven decades of medical research have given proof positive that heart disease can be reversed. In fact a bold proclamation was made by the editors of CV [Cardiovascular] *Review* in 1981 when they wrote: "It is conceivable that regression therapy might replace bypass surgery in many patients." When a professional journal makes such a statement, it is usually a sign of things to come.

So the question is not whether heart disease can be reversed, but *when* to start reversing heart disease. The answer to that is, *right now.* It doesn't matter if you are old or young, or even if you have had heart surgery or are about to have it. It is never too late or too early to prevent and modify atherosclerosis. The reversal diet program has a positive effect upon heart disease at any stage, although I believe, as do most of my colleagues, that treating atherosclerosis before it develops is much more effective and easier than treating it after coronary arteries are blocked. Nonetheless, if there are signs of atherosclerosis, research shows us that "newer" blockages reverse more quickly and more completely than "old" lesions, which means the earlier a program like this is started, the better.

The data on heart disease clearly show that you should start a reversal program as soon as possible. And while you are at it, encourage your spouse to begin such a program and even your children. The reason for this is simple: children learn from their parents. Or, as one of my colleagues says: "Healthy parents have healthy children, who have healthy dogs."

And, although heart disease usually progresses most rapidly between the ages of twenty and forty, it has its roots in childhood. Dr. Gerald Berenson, director of the Bogalusa (Louisiana) Heart Study, has accumulated some sobering facts from examining the heart health of 10,000 children in this southern town. He says levels of LDL cholesterol can be used to predict which children will have high cholesterol by the time they are six *months* old.

The Bogalusa study and the research of many others clearly show that heart disease begins in childhood. Elevated cholesterol levels in children mean even higher cholesterol levels as children mature toward adulthood. In a study in Muscatine, Iowa, Dr. Ronald Lauer proved this by testing 2,446 children at ages eight to eighteen and later retesting them at ages twenty to thirty. He found that of children with "high" cholesterol levels (greater than the 90th percentile) 43 percent were found to have equally high levels as twenty- to thirty-year-olds, 62 percent had levels greater than the 75th percentile, and 81 percent had levels greater than the 50th percentile. He found that a child with a blood-cholesterol level above 170 mg/dl is much more likely to have a level above 240 mg/dl as an adult. That is the main reason why it is important to screen children for elevated cholesterol levels from the time they are three years old.

Why so young? Research has shown that about 25 percent of American children have cholesterol levels that are too high—170 mg/dl or above—and about 5 percent have levels 200 mg/dl or higher.

Children should also have their blood pressure checked annually from the age of three, since hypertension begins to show itself at that tender age, especially in black children. As with cholesterol levels, elevated blood pressure in children is an indication that they are likely to have elevated blood pressure when they become adults.

The reversal diet program "immunizes" you or your child against later heart disease. It does this by teaching the life-style habits that prevent atherosclerosis. Because of that one factor alone, I recommend the reversal diet for children and adolescents regardless of their cholesterol levels. I make this recommendation because, as famed researcher Dr. Irvine H. Page commented in a speech, "good food habits should be learned while you are young. The food pattern available to most children and college youth is almost beyond belief—a high salt, high fat, high cholesterol diet irregularly wolfed down in the form of candy bars, fatty hamburgers or wieners and snacks. . . . We could do no worse, and this in part is due to home education and commercial enterprise."

Is it ever too late in your life to go on the reversal diet program? Not as far as I or the research data are concerned. The reversal diet program has its greatest effect upon people in their thirties to fifties. On the average, those are the years in which atherosclerosis progresses most quickly in men. But atherosclerosis happens to women, too. Their rate of coronary atherosclerosis catches up with that of men at age sixty-five.

A disease of multiple causes—which heart disease is—responds best to programs of multiple intervention. The reversal diet program can extend your life by attacking heart disease from all sides. Look at the effects of reducing cholesterol alone: several studies around the world have examined what happens to your chances of getting coronary heart disease when cholesterol is lowered. The results have consistently shown that for every 1 percent drop in cholesterol, there is a 2 percent decrease in the risk of coronary heart disease. The same is true for people who have already suffered one heart attack. For every 1 percent drop in their blood cholesterol levels, there is a 2 percent decrease in the chance that they will have another heart attack.

I'm not saying you will live forever, but I am saying that you will pack more years into your life and more life into your years by following the reversal diet program. Its results won't be hidden and unfelt. In addition to having the satisfaction of changing those "silent" numbers like blood pressure and cholesterol levels, the reversal diet will give you the energy of a person who functions better.

One of the unexpected but highly appreciated benefits that has happened to heart-disease patients in my intervention program is the increase in the frequency and quality of sexual activity.

You will realize something else, too. With the reversal diet program you will practice all things in moderation, but on the whole there is little you will miss.

Using This Book

The aim of this book is to show you how to alter the factors that contribute to heart disease yourself, without drugs if possible. I will explain how to do that in Chapter 2 by giving you a set of important goals to reach. As you will see, heart disease isn't necessarily caused by a single factor like elevated cholesterol. It is most often a combination of risk factors that lead to the buildup and accumulation of those blockages known as atherosclerosis. Consequently, the program I recommend also includes multiple risk-factor intervention—as mentioned earlier, diet, exercise, and other life-style changes.

After reading the reversal goals in Chapter 2 and then determining your reversal profile in Chapter 3, read the rest of the book to learn how to alter the factors that improve your chances of reversing heart disease. I think you will be amazed and pleasantly surprised at how easy it is to fit this program into your life. And I know you will be happy with the results.

THE
REVERSAL
DIET
PROGRAM

Eating,
Moving,
Thinking Your
Way to a
Healthier Heart

2

It is important to realize that heart disease is rarely caused by just one factor. If there is one thing cardiovascular research has taught us, it is that people with heart disease almost always have at least two of the following risk factors:

1. Maleness
2. *Increased* amounts of cholesterol in the blood (over 200 mg/dl)
3. High blood pressure (over 140/90)
4. Tobacco use
5. Diabetes or elevated blood-sugar levels
6. Excess body fat
7. A family history of premature vascular disease, heart disease, stroke, diabetes, or gout (in 60 percent of the subjects)
8. Abnormalities in electrocardiogram (EKG)
9. Reduced vital capacity
10. Stocky body build
11. A general lack of physical fitness

It is the many possible combinations of these factors that make the disease so complex. You might think that simply reducing your cholesterol level without achieving any of the other reversal goals will make you immune to coronary heart disease. That is no more true than the mistaken belief of one California pathologist who reported that completing a marathon, regardless of the time taken, grants you immunity from heart disease! No one thing appears to do that.

Heart disease is usually caused by a cluster of these risk factors—known as a *coronary constellation*—which act in concert to create the buildup of atherosclerosis.

The beauty of the reversal diet program is that it attacks *all* the factors that cause heart disease, not just one. It doesn't rely strictly upon dietary concerns, although the type of food you eat is the backbone of the program. The risk factors listed above can be eliminated or nullified by reaching these seven goals:

- **A total serum cholesterol of 200 mg/dl or less, LDL cholesterol of 130 mg/dl or less, with a total cholesterol/HDL ratio of 3.5 to 1 or less**
- **Normal blood pressure**
- **Regular exercise to improve fitness**
- **Body weight within 5 percent of normal**
- **Stress that doesn't result in strain-ful living**
- **No tobacco—period!**
- **Normal blood-sugar levels**

In this chapter I present the research that shows why these seven goals of the reversal program are important. It is very clear from the research that by reaching these goals you can turn your numbers around and let your body's own healing process begin.

There is little question that a low-blood-serum-cholesterol level—particularly LDL cholesterol—is the cornerstone of any program that hopes to stop or reverse the progression of atherosclerosis. But just "curing cholesterol" won't necessarily cure heart disease. Decades of research have shown that proper diet, no tobacco, safe blood pressure, lean body weight, and adequate exercise have profound effects upon the health of the heart, too.

Reversing heart disease is a war on many fronts. For example, if a person has high serum cholesterol, hypertension, and smokes, the "standard" risk of developing heart disease increases not just three times, but between nine and ten times. There can be risk of heart disease even if serum cholesterol levels aren't elevated. That is why the reversal diet program changes or nullifies all the risk factors, not just one or two.

Once you understand this principle, the next step is to apply this newfound knowledge to your own situation. You will take this step in Chapter 3 by compiling your own Reversal Profile, a personal medical record that shows you the "before and after" effects of the program.

This profile lets you take control of your health through two periods of self-observation. During the first period you keep track of your current cholesterol levels and the ratio of HDL to total cholesterol, as well as blood pressure, body weight, amount of exercise, and every scrap of food you eat.

The first period of observation will most likely reveal that some of your numbers are not within those called for in the reversal goals.

Those are obviously the numbers you will want to improve in this program.

The second period of self-observation should take place three months later. By then you will have read the book and will have made some life-style changes that the book recommends. The second period of self-observation will show the progress you will have made in reaching your reversal numbers. I think you will be amazed at how few life-style habits you will have to change to reap enormous health benefits. In fact, the changes are usually so easy to make that many patients who go on this program wonder why they haven't been on it all along.

When Will Reversal Take Place?

If you follow the advice in the rest of the book, the second period of observation in three months should find all of your numbers well within the reversal goals.

Then, you might wonder, *when will I begin reversing heart disease?* The data from years of research and my own personal observations indicate that you will begin reversing heart disease and your risk of heart disease within a few weeks.

After following the reversal diet program for six weeks, you will begin to lose weight and become more active. By virtue of that increased activity and weight loss, your heart will begin to function better and you will have much more energy. In addition, people who lose weight and become more active generally have less depression. So, if you have been under a cloud of depression or feeling just a touch of "the blues," those feelings should diminish substantially with the improvement in function that you will find in the early weeks of the reversal diet program.

Functional reversal is a beneficial spiral that feeds on itself. Weight loss and improved fitness lead to a better outlook which leads in turn to more weight loss and a more improved level of fitness.

These are the short-term benefits of the reversal diet program. They will motivate you so that you can receive the program's most important benefit—actual physiological reversal of blockage.

When will physiological reversal take place? Research shows that it takes anywhere from six months to five years, depending upon the age and progression of the atherosclerosis and the vigor with which you follow the reversal diet program. Reversal also depends upon whether the blockage has caused heart disease that is symptomatic, that is, whether blockage has progressed to the point where you have chest pains that have been diagnosed by a doctor as *ischemia,* or lack of blood flow to the heart muscle. These blockages usually take longer to reverse than the ones that haven't built up enough to cause pain. After examining data from more than a dozen regression studies, Dr. M. René Malinow, a noted researcher in the field of reversal, said that "reversal may be more common in persons without clinical indications." This means simply that reversal programs are more effective if started before blockage causes pain or electrocardiographic (EKG) changes.

Research published in *The Lancet,* a prestigious British medical journal, proved that early intervention is the most effective kind. The researchers, Dr. A. G. Olsson and colleagues, selected five patients who had high cholesterol levels but no symptoms of heart disease. That way they could examine the effects of a reversal diet on early atherosclerotic lesions.

Medicine and diet were used to lower total cholesterol and raise the amount of HDL. Angiograms taken before and after the cholesterol levels were altered revealed regression of atherosclerosis in the femoral arteries of all five patients.

This research shows that early reversal of heart disease is much more effective than waiting until symptoms manifest themselves. Or, as some wise person said: "An ounce of prevention is worth a pound of cure."

But that doesn't mean reversal doesn't occur when heart disease has progressed further; it just takes longer and is more difficult to achieve. Still it can be done. Dr. David Blankenhorn, in a *Cardiology Board Review* article on atherosclerosis regression, points out that mortality-based clinical trials, those that measure death rate in a given population, have shown lower death rates in older populations and therefore "provide indirect evidence for atherosclerotic regression." Direct evidence would be angiograms and the like.

Blankenhorn points to the Coronary Drug Project as an example of one such study. In that study, 8,341 men aged thirty to sixty-four years who had recovered from one or more heart attacks had their cholesterol levels lowered with drugs. Because all the study subjects had experienced at least one heart attack, it can be assumed that their lesions had been growing for some time. After six years of treatment, the patients whose cholesterol had been lowered by the drug niacin had less mortality than the other groups in the study. This reduced mortality is indirect evidence that regression had taken place.

Although lower cholesterol levels alone can reverse heart disease, some impressive examples of reversal have come from patients who use diets supplemented by other less quantifiable activities such as stretching, relaxation, meditation and yoga.

One of the most impressive studies of the effects of such life-style change without medication on coronary atherosclerosis is the study currently being conducted by Dr. Dean Ornish at the University of California at San Francisco School of Medicine that I mentioned in Chapter 1. To date Dr. Ornish and his colleagues have put twenty-nine patients with coronary artery disease on a reversal diet program that involves a reduction of fat and cholesterol in their diet, mild exercise, stress management, and smoking cessation. After only one year, this drug-free life-style program resulted in a nearly 4 percent reduction in the size of the lesions as shown by angiography and coronary blood flow to the heart muscle.

There are many other studies that point to the same conclusion: heart disease can be reversed. They all indicate roughly the same time frame, too: six months to five years.

An All-Purpose Program

The reversal diet program not only reverses heart disease, but also greatly reduces the chances of contracting other diseases and conditions that are caused by a Western diet. This subject was researched in depth by Dr. Denis Burkitt, a member of the London Medical Research Council. By comparing Third World and Western diets, he demonstrated a link between low-fiber intake and high incidence of ten medical conditions that are prevalent in the United States. He found that as fiber intake increases (as it does in the reversal diet program), the chances of contracting these conditions decrease. I am impressed that the diets to control or prevent atherosclerosis and to prevent cancer of the colon are almost identical.

Table 1 compares the effect of Western and Third World diets upon the health of their respective populations.

Table 1. COMPARISON OF WESTERN AND THIRD WORLD DISEASES

Condition	United States (High-Risk Diet)	Africa (Low-Risk Diet)
Ischemic heart disease	Responsible for one-third of all deaths	Virtually unknown; incidence beginning to increase slowly in large cities
Appendicitis	Most frequent of abdominal emergencies	Virtually unknown in rural areas; incidence beginning to increase in more Westernized communities
Diverticular disease	Most common disease of colon	Almost unknown
Gallstones	Present in some 10% of adult population	Exceedingly rare
Varicose veins	Present in over 10% of adult population	Present in probably under 0.1% of those living in traditional manner; increasing with adoption of Western customs
Deep-vein thrombosis and resultant pulmonary embolism	Hospital patients at high risk	Very rare
Hiatus hernia	Demonstrable in nearly half of population over 50 years old	Almost unknown
Hemorrhoids	Demonstrable in nearly half of population over 50 years old	Rare or very rare, according to degee of Westernization
Cancer of colon and rectum	Second only to lung cancer as cause of death from neoplasms	Rare
Obesity	Nearly half of adult population markedly overweight	Rare among those living wholly on traditional diets; increasingly common with urbanization and adoption of Western foods

Source: D. P. Burkitt, "Etiology and Prevention of Colorectal Cancer," *Hospital Practice*, February 1974.

Decades of working as a surgeon and a preventive-medicine practitioner in Africa have led Burkitt to the conclusion that surgery is wonderful, but prevention is better.

Let's examine the seven goals of the Reversal Diet in more detail.

GOAL 1: To Reduce Total Cholesterol to below 200 mg/dl and LDL Cholesterol below 130 mg/dl, (with a Total Cholesterol/HDL Ratio of 3.5)

When Dr. N. N. Anitschkow said nearly fifty years ago that "without cholesterol there is no atherosclerosis," he was very nearly right. Cholesterol is the main building block of atherosclerosis, which is why most of this book is devoted to simple and pleasant ways of reducing blood-cholesterol levels and controlling blood cholesterol over the long term. The measures you are about to take in the reversal diet program lower serum cholesterol and raise the level of "good" HDL cholesterol.

Study after study has shown strong links between high serum-cholesterol levels and high rates of heart disease. Just how much effect cholesterol levels have on heart disease is clear from data from the Framingham Study, which show that men with an average blood-cholesterol level of 260 experience heart attacks three times as often as men with levels below 195 mg/dl.

In a thirty-year follow-up examination of the Framingham data, cardiovascular deaths rose 9 percent in men and women under the age of fifty for every 10-milligram rise in serum cholesterol. And other studies show a 2 percent reduction in heart disease risk for every 1 percent reduction in total cholesterol levels.

Reducing cholesterol does more than stop the buildup. Research shows that a lowering of serum cholesterol reduces the actual size of an atherosclerotic lesion.

Serum cholesterol can be reduced in three ways:

• **Decrease intake:** The average American diet contains about 600 milligrams of cholesterol per day, twice the amount recommended by the American Heart Association.

By eliminating a few foods, such as eggs, which contain about 275 milligrams of cholesterol each, and using an egg substitute, people who are heavy egg eaters could probably bring their serum-cholesterol levels closer to the reversal range of 200 mg/dl and stop or at least slow the progression of heart disease. Reducing total fat intake to 30 percent, with 10 percent being from saturated fat, will likely lead to lower serum cholesterol.

• *Increase cholesterol loss:* This can be done by exercising regularly, by using cholesterol-lowering medication and/or eating foods that are high in fiber. Exercise at moderate levels increases the consumption of fat stores, lowering triglycerides and total cholesterol and elevating HDL cholesterol.

If the fiber happens to be soluble, for example, oat bran or some fruits such as apples, it has the added effect of sticking to cholesterol in the bile and passing this substance from your body via your stools. This makes it more effective in reducing serum-cholesterol levels than the insoluble fiber found in vegetables and wheat products, which cannot be broken down in the intestines by digestive juices. In fact, consuming two ounces of soluble fiber each day has been shown to reduce cholesterol levels in people by 5 to 10 percent. Recent research has emphasized that oat bran is not superior to fiber in other cereals, but that both are effective because they supplant saturated fats in the diet.

• *Interfere with production:* Sometimes the liver produces much more cholesterol than the body needs for the production of important hormones and bile. There is a rare inherited disorder known as *familial hypercholesterolemia.* This problem can be detected in early childhood, but if left undetected it can often lead to death before the age of fifty.

If you have this disease, it may be necessary for you to use one of the drugs that interfere with enzyme production. Although these drugs are currently very expensive, they are very effective in reducing serum cholesterol. However, they produce side effects, such as constipation and abdominal cramps, in 5–6 percent of users or skeletal muscle changes in less than 1 in 100, that cause them to be discontinued in about 2 percent. Many patients prefer these drugs to the bile sequestrants, which are gritty, often unpleasant, and more constipative.

THE ROLE OF HDL

Recently, the type—and not just the amount—of cholesterol has also come under scrutiny. Too little of the "good" HDL (high-density lipoprotein) cholesterol has been implicated in high heart-disease rates in people with otherwise desirable serum-cholesterol levels. HDL cholesterol participates in reverse transport. Without sufficient amounts of HDL to attach to the "bad" LDL cholesterol and pull this harmful substance from the bloodstream, the atherosclerotic buildup can occur regardless of total blood-cholesterol levels.

The latest research showing that low HDL levels can lead to heart disease has been done at the Johns Hopkins Medical Centers in Baltimore, where 1,000 patients with cholesterol levels less than 200 mg/dl (well within the desirable range) had their coronary arteries examined by angiography. Of the 1,000 patients examined, 232 had coronary artery disease. Upon further examination the researchers found that the average HDL level of these patients was 35 milligrams. Such an HDL level translates into a 50 percent higher risk for heart disease than an HDL level of 45 milligrams.

More and more research is showing that high levels of the good HDL cholesterol and low amounts of LDL cholesterol in your blood often reverse atherosclerosis or stop its progression. Researchers have devised a simplified ratio for total cholesterol to HDL. It is figured by dividing total cholesterol by HDL. For example, a total serum-cholesterol count of 200 mg/dl, divided by an HDL count of 60, would equal a ratio of 3.3. A ratio of 3.5 or better is optimal. The total cholesterol/HDL ratio is usually calculated for you when your blood is tested.

Fortunately, exercising, reducing amounts of saturated fats and cholesterol, losing weight, and quitting cigarette smoking all lead to a rise in HDL levels.

CHOLESTEROL GOALS

• *A serum cholesterol under 200 mg/dl with a total cholesterol/ HDL ratio of approximately 3.5 or less:* In most of the reversal studies, the humans and animals examined achieved reversal or stopped the progression of their atherosclerotic lesions with cholesterol levels that didn't dip lower than 150. In fact, many of the subjects have had levels higher than 200, as in David Blankenhorn's studies, in which he successfully reversed the buildup in the femoral arteries of humans.

The "ideal" cholesterol level is not known. However, in societies with very little coronary heart disease, the serum-cholesterol level is about 150 mg/dl. This has led many researchers to believe that the target level for maximum reversal should be a cholesterol level of 150 mg/dl.

All the changes called for in the reversal diet program work to lower total cholesterol and improve the total cholesterol/HDL ratio.

GOAL 2: Achieve a Normal Blood Pressure of 140/90 or Better

High blood pressure can turn a little cholesterol problem into a big one. By increasing blood-flow pressure, this usually silent killer increases the buildup of cholesterol on the walls of arteries. The best guess is that the high pressure "cracks" the delicate lining of the arteries, forcing LDLs into the intima and speeding the buildup of atherosclerosis.

People with hypertension have heart disease three times as often as those without it. Even mild hypertension, such as blood pressure above 140/90, can double cardiovascular risk. And the risk of cardiovascular disease presented by hypertension is the same for women as for men.

Hypertension is a silent and scary problem that can go unnoticed, the way elevated cholesterol levels do. Recent studies have shown that only about 40 percent of patients with high blood pressure have been aware of their affliction. Of those, only 30 percent were under treatment, and 14 percent were found to be under "good control."

Your blood pressure can be raised by:

- Obesity
- A diet high in sodium
- Smoking
- Low levels of exercise if physically unfit
- A stressful life-style

Although drugs have long been the most common way of controlling blood pressure, studies are showing that they may not be the best way. In one such study, ninety-seven patients with mild hypertension were taken off medication and given nutritional counseling instead. In addition to showing a 5- to 10-pound weight loss over the four-year period of the study, almost 40 percent were able to stay off hypertension drugs and maintain normal blood pressure.

Since the reversal diet program calls for exercise and lower sodium intake, and encourages weight reduction, its effects upon hypertension should be even greater than those reported in the study mentioned above.

If your blood pressure is in the safe range already, congratulate yourself. You can interpret the reading your doctor gives you by comparing it to the guidelines below.

Table 2. BLOOD PRESSURE EVALUATION

Range (mm Hg)	Category
Diastolic blood pressure (lowest pressure; the bottom number in your reading)	
Below 85	Normal blood pressure
85 to 89	High normal
90 to 104	Mild hypertension
105 to 114	Moderate hypertension
Above 114	Severe hypertension
Systolic blood pressure (highest pressure)—when diastolic is below 90—	
Below 140	Normal blood pressure
140 to 159	Borderline isolated systolic hypertension
Above 159	Isolated systolic hypertension

Categories recommended by the 1988 Report of the Joint National Committee on Detection, Evaluation, and Treatment of High Blood Pressure in *Archives of Internal Medicine* 1988; 148: 1023–1038.

If you can't congratulate yourself, consult your physician and let him know that you want to change your numbers by trying the drug-free reversal diet program. The diet, exercise, and stress-reduction advice contained in these pages should lower most blood pressures.

If this drug-free attempt fails to lower blood pressure enough, there are many effective antihypertension drugs on the market that will usually do the job. However, it is best to avoid them if possible, since all of them have side effects and some even raise serum cholesterol while lowering blood pressure.

GOAL 3: Burn at Least 150 to 300 Calories per Day with Heart-Strengthening Exercise

Exercise is good for you. That fact becomes clearer with every new study. Not only does it promote longer life, but it also leads to a better quality of life. Much of this is due to its profound effects upon the heart and circulatory system. The simplest explanation for this is that much of the body is made of muscle, and to stay strong and healthy muscle has to be used.

A study conducted at the Institute for Aerobic Research in Dallas best illustrates this point. Between 1970 and 1981, 13,000 men and 4,000 women with an average age in the low forties were put on exercise programs. Researchers found that those who failed to continue their exercise programs increased their chances of premature death two to three times.

Other research has shown that the more calories you expend each week, the less are your chances of dying from a heart attack. For example, people who run or walk twenty miles a week burn approximately 2,000 calories in exercise. Their rate of heart attack is 64 percent lower than that of people who expend 500 calories a week in exercise.

Exercise alone has been shown to halt the progression of atherosclerosis in men with coronary artery disease. A total of 104 men with heart disease were put on carefully monitored exercise programs and given angiograms at the beginning of the study and again twenty months later. The increase in exercise was associated with stopping the progression of arterial disease in many of the subjects. This study demonstrates the healing power of exercise alone, since it didn't even combine exercise with diet and the other reversal interventions!

There are many reasons why exercise has such a profound effect upon the body and the cardiovascular system in particular. Here are a few of them:

• *Exercise dissolves blood clots:* Do you remember that clot-forming molecule fibrinogen mentioned in Chapter 1? Remember how it forms over rough spots on the top of an atheroma and together with blood platelets forms a blood clot?

Exercise inspires the production of an enzyme called fibrinolysin, or *fibrin dissolver.* It actually has the function of dissolving blood clots and "thinning" the blood so the blood clots more slowly and flows more freely.

Thus, in addition to making the blood flow better, which exercisers need, the increased level of fibrinolysin also serves to dissolve clots that might be present in the arteries.

That increased fibrinolysin level helps reduce heart-disease risk. A study conducted by Dr. Nirmal Sarkas and published in the British publication *Nature* showed that the blood from people with "normal" circulation was able to dissolve 95 percent of a clot within twenty-four hours. Blood from people with atherosclerosis, on the other hand, was able to dissolve only 64 percent of the clot during the same time. Exercise increases the blood's clot-dissolving properties.

• *Exercise increases HDL, the good cholesterol:* Exercise increases the amount of HDL cholesterol in the bloodstream, the "scavengers" that work to clear the "bad" LDLs from the body. Why is this? Speculation has it that HDL cholesterol is synthesized from fat food particles known as chlyomicrons instead of in the liver where LDLs are produced. This synthesis takes place because exercise stimulates production of an enzyme that converts chlyomicrons into HDL.

Studies have shown that a particle of HDL usually lasts about five days in the bloodstream before being passed from the body. It is for this reason that *regular* exercise is needed to keep HDL levels elevated.

• *Exercise reduces blood pressure:* Regular aerobic exercise—activities such as jogging, brisk walking, swimming, cycling, cross-country skiing—have been shown to decrease blood pressure.

In the Harvard Alumni study, for example, in which the life-style habits of 16,936 graduates of that Ivy League school were studied for sixteen years, the risk of developing high blood pressure was much lower for the physically active. Even among "heavyweights" (men 25 percent or more overweight for their height), the risk of developing hypertension was one-fourth less when they participated in two hours per week of vigorous activity.

• *Exercise promotes healthy weight loss:* Exercise combined with dieting reduces the amount of body fat while increasing muscle. On the other hand, dieting without exercise promotes the loss of both fat and muscle. So if you are an inactive dieter, you might lose ten pounds, but because of physical inactivity, much of what is lost will be muscle along with fat. Since muscle burns fat as fuel, the continued loss of muscle through improper dieting will make it harder to lose weight because the body's fuel-burning capacity will be dwindling. This relative rise in body fat will also make you less healthy.

Exercise alone with no change in diet will inspire weight loss, too. For example, I once treated a lawyer who was an overweight 246 pounds. By walking one hour a day, he burned an average of 360 calories per session and lost 40 pounds by the end of the year. In addition, he lowered his blood pressure, reduced his serum cholesterol, and improved his heart function—all that benefit from one simple life-style change.

• *Exercise improves heart function:* Exercise improves your heart's pumping ability and increases stroke volume, the amount of blood it can push with each beat. This increased efficiency slows the heart rate, which means your heart muscle doesn't need as much oxygen for a given level of effort. It isn't uncommon for a trained athlete to have a resting pulse rate of around 40 beats per minute (bpm), whereas an untrained person might have a resting pulse rate in the range of 70 bpm. The athlete's heart is doing the same job more efficiently.

Exercise also causes an increase in oxidative enzymes in the exercised muscle allowing them to extract and utilize more oxygen from the passage of blood.

Improved heart function is one way in which the reversal diet program can reverse physiological aging. By slowing heart rate and improving oxygen capacity, your heart actually functions as it did when it was younger. In my studies, I have exercise-trained sixty-year-old heart patients and made their hearts as strong as those of normal forty-year-olds.

Add to all of these benefits the fact that exercise usually makes you a happier person, less depressed and more confident, and you have something that would probably be the best-selling drug if it were in pill form. Fortunately, however, it is free. But unfortunately it doesn't get used enough. According to a 1984 survey by the Centers for Disease Control, only 9 percent of Americans exercise enough to meet minimum standards. The reversal diet program will make you one of those self-chosen few.

EXERCISE GOALS

• *Burn at least 150 to 300 calories a day in exercise:* Although you can burn your calories any way you choose, there is added benefit from vigorous exercise. That is why I recommend following the American College of Sports Medicine (ACSM) guidelines, which recommend exercise three days a week, twenty minutes a session.

The ACSM released exercise guidelines in 1980 so people would know how much exercise was enough. I was one of the doctors involved in compiling that consensus report. We examined more than ninety medical studies to determine the amount of exercise needed to improve cardiovascular function without over- or underdoing it.

Our results were based on solid medical science, which is why I recommend them here. These are minimum requirements for exercise, the least you should do to ensure the benefits outlined above.

• *Exercise at least three days a week:* Every other day is the preferred schedule. That gives you a day in between to recover and also spreads out the effects of training to make exercise easier.

• *Exercise at least 20 to 30 minutes per session:* Twenty to thirty minutes of exercise was considered to be the minimum amount of sustained and vigorous movement necessary to garner the rewards of aerobic exercise. Add to this a 5- to 10-minute warmup and an equal period to cool down.

• *Exercise at 60 to 90 percent of your maximum heart rate:* Elevating heart rate is necessary to make exercise aerobic. But what should be your target heart rate? The ACSM says that 60 to 90 percent of your maximum heart rate (obtained on a treadmill or bicycle ergometer) for at least twenty minutes fits the definition of aerobic.

To figure target heart rate, follow this equation: 220 minus your age in years, multiplied by 0.60 to 0.90 = target heart rate.

For example, here's the *theoretical minimal target training heart rate* for a healthy forty-five-year-old man: $220 - 45 = 175 \times 0.60 = 105$ beats per minute. *Maximal* 158 bpm. However if this man was able to attain a heart rate of only 160 bpm on a treadmill test, the range of his training heart rate would be 96 to 144 ($0.60 \times 160 = 96$; $0.90 \times 160 = 144$).

It is better that your training heart rate be obtained from your response during an exercise test rather than relying upon the theoretical maximal heart rate, because of individual variations.

• *In addition to following the ACSM guidelines, get random exercise whenever you can:* With exercise, as with saving money, every little bit helps. In a world dominated by cars and computers, it is easy to spend more time on your rear end than on your feet. In the sit-down environment in which most of us live it is necessary to *look* for ways to get exercise.

Research shows that random exercise pays off. The Harvard Alumni study demonstrates the value of calories burned in *any* endeavor, including "background" exercise such as climbing stairs and mowing the lawn. The researchers found that this seemingly benign extra effort contributes to overall health and life expectancy. So take the stairs instead of the escalator when you can. The extra effort will cost you about eight calories per minute while building muscle and stamina.

Although you should certainly see a physician before starting any exercise program, you should keep something else in mind, too: many more people are adversely affected by lack of exercise than by too much exercise. And don't be afraid to go beyond these recommendations.

The further magic of exercise is covered in Chapter 8.

GOAL 4: Maintain a Normal Body Weight

An obese person is nearly three times more likely to get heart disease or die from it than a person with normal body weight.

The reversal diet calls for a body weight within 5 percent of normal as determined by the Height/Weight Tables devised in 1959 by the Metropolitan Life Insurance Company.

There are more recent Metropolitan tables, but in our opinion and that of others, they allow a person to be too heavy. The most recent controversy involving the "heavier" tables comes from a survey of 115,886 women to see how extra weight affects their risk of heart disease.

The study, conducted at Boston's Brigham and Women's Hospital, found that almost any extra weight increases risk of heart disease for women (5 to 14 percent above Metropolitan's ideal weight increased risk of heat disease by 30 percent, 15 to 29 percent equalled an 80 percent increase in risk).

"We were very surprised that the risk of heart disease was high for women who were only mildly overweight," Dr. JoAnn Manson, the study's chief author, told the *Wall Street Journal*. "I think if anything, the ideal weight on the tables should be revised downward."

The study suggested that 40 percent of all heart disease in women is due to being overweight, even slightly.

This study is among the reasons we are using the lighter tables.

By reaching the other six goals and following the diet information in the rest of the book, your weight should reduce to normal as your other numbers come into the reversal range.

Obesity refers to an excessive amount of fat below the skin and in the abdominal cavity. Ideally body fat can be *measured precisely* by weighing under water, and can be *estimated* by measuring the thickness of several skinfolds—the so-called pinch test. For men, normal body fat is 10 to 15 percent, overweight 20 to 25 percent, and obese more than 25 percent body fat. For women, the normal range is 20 to 25 percent, overweight 30 to 35 percent, and obese more than 35 percent body fat. Most people rely on a less accurate, but still highly valuable, method of relating body height to body weight, taking into account the body frame: small, medium, and large.

Table 3.   HEIGHT/WEIGHT TABLES

Normal Weights
(When Weighed with Indoor Clothing and Shoes)

Height	Small Frame (lbs)	Medium Frame (lbs)	Large Frame (lbs)
Men			
5'2"	112–120	118–129	126–141
5'3"	115–123	121–133	129–144
5'4"	118–126	124–136	132–148
5'5"	121–129	127–139	135–152
5'6"	124–133	130–143	138–156
5'7"	128–137	134–147	142–161
5'8"	132–141	138–152	147–166
5'9"	136–145	142–156	151–170
5'10"	140–150	146–160	155–174
5'11"	144–154	150–165	159–179
6'0"	148–158	154–170	164–184
6'1"	152–162	158–175	168–189
6'2"	158–167	162–180	173–194
6'3"	160–171	167–185	178–199
6'4"	164–175	172–190	182–204

Height	Normal Weights (When Weighed with Indoor Clothing and Shoes)		
	Small Frame (lbs)	Medium Frame (lbs)	Large Frame (lbs)
Women			
4'10"	92–98	96–107	104–119
4'11"	94–101	98–110	106–122
5'0"	96–104	101–113	109–125
5'1"	99–107	104–116	112–128
5'2"	102–110	107–119	115–131
5'3"	105–113	110–122	118–134
5'4"	108–116	113–126	121–138
5'5"	111–119	116–130	125–142
5'6"	114–123	120–135	129–146
5'7"	118–127	124–139	133–150
5'8"	122–131	128–143	137–154
5'9"	126–135	132–147	141–158
5'10"	130–140	136–151	145–163
5'11"	134–144	140–155	149–168
6'0"	138–148	144–159	153–173

Source: Metropolitan Life Insurance Company.

GOAL 5: De-Stress Your Life

You know stress when you are experiencing it, but it's usually difficult to define. A famous eighteenth-century surgeon named John Hunter certainly knew it when it happened. He had a touchy case of angina pectoris, chest pains caused by reduced blood flow to the heart, which flared up when he was angry. He was rumored to have said: "My life is in the hands of any rascal who chooses to annoy or tease me." That proved to be prophetic. Hunter later died from a heart attack that occurred during an argument at a hospital staff meeting.

Since then, stress has been blamed for many conditions of the heart. Some of this blame is warranted and some is not.

For instance, there is solid research to show that periods of job stress, frustration, and fear do cause a rise in cholesterol levels. In one study conducted at Mount Zion Medical Center in San Francisco, accountants were shown to have higher blood cholesterol during the two weeks before the income-tax filing deadline on April 15 than during February or March, when their job loads were lower. The same trend has been shown in medical students before taking exams.

Adrenaline is one possible culprit in this stress-related rise in serum cholesterol. When a stressful event occurs, the body prepares itself for "fight or flight," the response mechanism that allowed our cavemen ancestors to fight a small animal or run from a large one effectively.

The perception, or the symbolic significance of nonphysical stresses, such as decisions, time deadlines, interpersonal relationships, arguments, and the responses to them may be potentially harmful.

These days few stressful situations call for fleeing or fighting, but the body responds by releasing adrenaline anyway. So when you find yourself in a difficult situation—trying to explain a lost account to your boss or hoping that the freeway traffic will start moving so you can make it on time to an important appointment—the adrenaline goes to work in your body, not knowing that you just can't pick up and run.

It causes a release of fatty acids into your bloodstream that your caveman ancestors would have used as quick fuel. But without physical activity these fats just flow through your body.

At moments of stress a hormone called *cortisol* is also excreted by the adrenal gland. It elevates cholesterol, but you can't burn cholesterol as fuel without physical movement. So at times of stress, cholesterol circulates in the bloodstream.

The adrenaline is also tensing your muscles, raising blood pressure, and squeezing down on your arteries. More of the blood's clotting factors are floating around, making the chance of a clot much greater. That's fine if a saber-toothed tiger is on the prowl. But here in the modern jungle of the twentieth century, we don't often get to run from our problems. We are forced to deal with them in a civilized (i.e., a nonphysical) manner.

But is all stress bad? Certainly not. Stress is necessary for an organism to grow and improve. In fact some people thrive on it.

That is the basic flaw in the assumption that "Type A's" are more prone to a heart attack than "Type B's." The assumption of cardiologists Meyer Friedman and Ray Rosenman in the 1970s was that Type A behavior patterns marked by a sense of time urgency, aggressiveness, hostility, ambition, drive, and competitiveness would lead to a greater likelihood of heart disease.

What they failed to account for was a factor known as "symbolic interpretation of stress." Although researchers can quantify many stressful factors, they can't tell what will actually be stressful to a particular individual. So while "on paper" a situation might appear stressful, in reality a person might find the situation to his or her liking. I discovered this fact with my own studies.

At the same time Friedman and Rosenman were formulating their theories on Type A personalities, I was doing studies on two groups that fit into that "Type A" very nicely: trial attorneys and surgeons. My research revealed that although the stresses of trial work and surgery could be quantifiable, the responses of the people within each of these two groups varied considerably. I knew their internal responses because I had hooked them up to a device called a Holter Monitor that would allow me to record their heart rates and electrocardiograms over a twenty-four-hour period.

Some of the lawyers and surgeons who seemed stressed on the outside really weren't stressed internally. The opposite was true also. Some who appeared to be cool as cucumbers responded with high heart rates and blood pressure. Eventually, we could even tell which of the surgeons would leave surgery for teaching positions or have a higher rate of heart disease (or both) by the way they responded to the stresses of their job. They were the ones who had a higher heart-rate response during surgery, higher systolic and diastolic blood pressure, more depression, and lower self-esteem and were physically less fit. And they repressed their feelings. Or as the psychologist on one study said: "They felt without acting and acted without feeling."

The research showed that stress output is not the same as stress input: the stress may be the same, but the people respond differently. It wasn't Type A that was a risk factor for heart disease, but the *response* of the Type A personality. It became clear that the fast-moving top executive who had to make snap decisions were actually living longer than others in their age groups.

For instance a follow-up look at Type A male patients in the Western Collaborative Group Study of Friedman and Rosenman showed that they were outliving the "cooler" Type B patients.

With additional research the Type A hypothesis changed to what it is now: the generally accepted belief that "hostile" Type A's run a higher risk of heart disease. By themselves such factors as ambition, drive, aggressiveness, competitiveness, and a sense of time urgency might not contribute to heart disease at all.

This pocket synopsis shows how difficult stress is to quantify. We can't attach numbers to stress levels the way we can to blood-cholesterol levels because people respond very differently to stressors. Stress is something that has to be assessed one person at a time. Let me give you an example:

A patient in one of my studies was depressed and feeling stressed in his life. Although it is common for some heart-disease patients to feel depressed as a result of their illness, his depression was much worse than it should have been. I spoke to him and found that before his heart problems developed he had been in charge of fifteen people at the factory where he worked. But because of his heart attack, his boss did him a "favor" and reduced the number of people under him to six. Although he had lost no income, he felt a loss of status and was showing signs of strain.

The psychiatrist on this study who was from India said, "In my country, we get depressed like this after running out of food for two or three days."

That was it exactly! He was starving—starving for self-esteem. Although the managers thought they were reducing this man's stress by cutting back on his workload, they were actually making his life more stressful. Instead of doing my patient a favor, the boss at this factory was actually starving him of his nourishment of authority. It was a response that was entirely different from the one many would have predicted.

Maybe it's not stress that is the problem, but strain. After all, stress is simply a force applied to an object. Strain is what happens when that force is more than the object can bear.

Do you know these feelings? These are the symptoms of responses to stress. Not only are these symptoms hard on your cardiovascular system, but they can also lead you to behaviors that are harmful to your heart in other ways.

In our society, for example, food is a source of comfort for many people. When faced with a stressful situation, many of you head for a well-stocked refrigerator where you temporarily drown stress (and the reversal diet) with between-meal snacks. Some of you might smoke cigarettes in response to stress. Others might become lethargic and inactive, opting to sit and sulk rather than stand and fight stress with a hearty walk around the block. Stress can launch a host of behaviors that promote heart disease. If these stresses happen to make you

hostile, research shows that you are more likely to smoke more cigarettes, drink more alcohol, and even eat more.

The diet and exercise advice in the reversal diet program will help
negate the stresses of "strain-ful" living. By following the guidelines
of this book, especially those relating to exercise, you will "burn" the
products of stress. Also, you will have feelings of greater control,
which always lower stress and strain levels.

STRESS AND STRAIN GOALS

• *Learn to recognize negative stresses in your life and cope with
them:* I know this recommendation is almost as amorphous as defining
stress itself. But physical stress is usually an individually interpreted
response that requires individual diagnosis. When you feel "stress,"
recognize it for what it is. Try to determine its importance and value
to you and decide on a type of action. Choose your remedy—action,
indifference, whatever you think appropriate. Think it over. Physical
activities like walking, jogging, wood chopping, gardening, or climbing the stairs at work often serve as "stress relievers."

Also learn to relax. There are many available programs that promote relaxation techniques, including meditation, classes at the
YMCA, YWCA, and other community facilities.

GOAL 6: Use No Tobacco

If I had to "choose my poison," an elevated cholesterol level or smoking cigarettes, I would opt for the higher cholesterol without a moment's hesitation.

Luckily we don't have to make hard health choices like that one.
But such a choice underscores the deadly nature of the cigarette. In
any form, be it filtered or full-strength, low tar or cool menthol,
cigarettes spell disaster for the human heart.

Just how bad cigarette smoking is can be shown by examining data
from the Multiple Risk Factor Intervention Trial (MR. FIT), a study
of 361,662 men. Researchers found that a smoker with a cholesterol
level under 181 mg/dl has the same risk of heart disease as a nonsmoker with a cholesterol level almost 60 points higher!

There are many factors that make smoking a high-risk proposition
for the heart. For instance:

- The inhalation of carbon monoxide forms a compound with hemoglobin (red blood cells) in which the oxygen is not available to the body. As a result the heart muscle starves for oxygen and weakens at rest and weakens even more with exercise.
- Nicotine in the cigarette stimulates the release of adrenaline, which causes blood vessels to squeeze down, restricting the blood flow and possibly causing damage to the delicate intima. This adrenaline in the bloodstream also mobilizes fat, which clouds the blood with fatty acids, making it even thicker. In fact, people who smoke theoretically should run a mile after each cigarette to burn up all of those fatty acids floating in their bloodstream.
- There is a rise in clotting factors such as fibrin and platelets, which greatly increases the chance that blood clots will form in areas that have atherosclerotic lesions.
- And, speaking of lesions, the tars in tobacco have mutagenic qualities that can cause them. Add to this the fact that cigarettes reduce the amount of "good" HDL cholesterol in most smokers and you have a risk factor that outweighs all others.

In addition to all the damage smoking does to the heart, it is often the *coup de grâce* in a heart attack. A smoker who has a heart attack is two to four times as likely to die from it than a nonsmoker, partly because the heart is starved for oxygen, a condition known as *ischemia*. A study conducted at the Brigham and Women's Hospital in Boston and published in the Journal of the American Medical Association compared twenty-one smokers with forty-one nonsmokers and found that patients with coronary artery disease who smoke have "significantly and substantially" more ischemia than their nonsmoking counterparts.

Even going smokeless with snuff is no solution. A study published in the *Annals of Internal Medicine* found that men who use snuff or chewing tobacco get the same amount of nicotine as cigarette smokers, enough to increase blood pressure and heart rate as much as if they were just like people using the real thing.

TOBACCO GOALS

• *Stop all use of tobacco:* This is a must for the reversal or prevention of heart disease. But saying it is easier than doing it. A 1989 Surgeon General's report on smoking says it can be a habit as tough to break as heroin addiction, which may account for the large number of people who can "quit anytime" and have, many times over.

If you plan to go on the reversal diet program, you must stop smoking. And because of its truly addictive nature, smokers usually need special help in kicking the habit. Luckily, there are many specialized clinics around the country that offer help in this difficult endeavor.

Although your heart and lungs will thank you immediately, research shows that it takes about ten years after a pack-a-day smoker quits for his or her risk of heart disease to be equal to that of someone who has never used tobacco. The reversal diet program can greatly improve your odds of avoiding heart problems, but only if you become an "ex"-smoker.

GOAL 7: Maintain Normal Blood-Sugar Levels

Getting food to the cells that need them is part of good nutrition. But this process is sometimes hampered by high blood-sugar levels, or diabetes.

Your body uses the energy of blood sugar in the form of glucose. In normal individuals, glucose leaves the bloodstream and enters cells with the help of insulin, which is produced in the pancreas. Without insulin, glucose builds up in the blood while surrounding tissues starve for its energy. Without glucose, muscles and organs are forced to use fat as an alternative source of energy. This fat is released into the bloodstream. If there is an overabundance of these fatty acids, they clog the arteries and create blockages.

There are two types of diabetes.

Type 1 diabetes is characterized by insufficient production of insulin and usually calls for insulin to be injected on a daily basis.

Type 2 is often genetic and is usually brought on by obesity. Type

2's can produce some insulin, but their ability to utilize glucose is impaired by genetic factors.

Few Type 2 diabetics require injectable insulin. Their disease can usually be controlled by diet (and I am referring here to the reversal diet) and by exercise. Sometimes oral medication is required.

The power of diet to control diabetes is dramatically illustrated by the results of the Chicago Coronary Prevention Evaluation Program that was conducted from 1958 to 1973. Program director Dr. Jeremiah Stamler encouraged 158 men who had two or more risk factors for heart disease to switch to a diet similar to the reversal diet. They lowered their saturated fat and cholesterol intake, ate slightly more polyunsaturated fats, and moderated their use of sugar and alcohol.

Every three months, Stamler had them complete a seven-day food diary like the one you will be keeping for this program. After 2 and 4 years, the diaries reflected a 50 percent reduction in dietary cholesterol intake, a one-third reduction in saturated fat intake, and an average intake of 600 calories less per day. Serum cholesterol dropped an average of 10 percent.

The ability to digest blood sugar as measured by glucose-tolerance tests mirrored the weight loss of these subjects. The men who lost the most weight showed the greatest reduction in blood-sugar levels.

It has been observed that a change in diet for the Type 2 diabetic reverses heart disease. This was the subject of a commentary by Dr. Timothy Leary, a Boston pathologist who studied heart disease in the 1930s:

"In connection with no other disease has there been such widespread experimentation in pathogenesis as was carried out in the feeding of diabetic diets [that were] high in fat, rich in cholesterol, in the decade 1920–30. The results were as definite as those obtained in the experimental rabbit. The human lesions were spectacular enough particularly in children. Moreover, the reverse procedure, a cutting down of fats in the diet, including cholesterol, resulted in a return to the status quo."

BLOOD-SUGAR GOALS

• *Keep sugar levels in line with age and weight:* Diabetes is often recognized by its symptoms: fatigue, increased thirst and hunger, and increased urination. If you have persistent symptoms like these, a blood-glucose test may be in order. You might want to have a glucose test anyway, just to be sure. Studies have shown that over half of the subjects who test positive for high blood sugar are completely unaware of its presence.

For healthy, normal men and women the range of blood glucose is between 80 to 105 mg/dl. However, many elderly subjects have fasting glucose levels higher than 120 mg/dl, and although they are not considered to be clinically diabetic, glucose tolerance may be abnormal because of age-related increased insulin resistance.

The Right Choices

The goals for reversing heart disease illustrate that it is usually a disease of life-style. And, as is the case with all diseases of life-style, your chance of having one of the million and a half heart attacks predicted to occur this year in America (or of having another) can be greatly reduced by making some life-style changes.

I don't mean to say that coronary heart disease is self-inflicted. That would imply that we are trying to hurt ourselves by the way we live. That is rarely true.

Generally speaking, life-styles are taught to us by our parents. The children of vegetarians grow up and become vegetarians just as meat-eating children remain carnivores. We tend to exercise as adults as we exercised as kids. And few people start smoking as adults. They usually start the habit as teenagers with the help of mom or dad.

So I dislike thinking of heart disease as self-inflicted, especially since we have had so much help choosing our life-styles throughout our lives.

But it is good to know that with heart disease—unlike some diseases—you have another chance. By achieving these seven goals you can reverse, stop, or at least slow its progression.

YOUR
REVERSAL
PROFILE

*Charting
Your
Course
through the
Seven Goals
of Reversal*

3

Before you begin to make changes to achieve the reversal goals, it is important to take an inventory of where you stand. After all, you can't change something if you don't know what you're changing. That is why you need your own Reversal Profile to see how you stack up against this program's goals.

The Reversal Profile consists essentially of your own medical records. To compile them you need to have two standard blood tests performed by your physician: a serum-cholesterol test that gives you total cholesterol as well as a total cholesterol/HDL ratio, and a reading of your blood-sugar levels. These tests should be done after a twelve- to fourteen-hour fast, which generally means you can have blood drawn in the morning, provided you skip breakfast.

I recommend seeing your physician for these tests. Although they are often available free or at low cost through community screening programs, the laboratory that your personal physician uses provides the consistent results that you will need when you repeat the tests in three months to complete your Reversal Profile Progress Report. Although community screenings are usually accurate, some of the equipment used may not be standardized to the National Cholesterol Education Program's recommendations. In fact you should not hesitate to ask your doctor questions about the accuracy of the laboratory's cholesterol measurements. If he asks why you are concerned, mention the 1985 study conducted by the College of American Pathologists showing that 47 percent of the 5,000 labs they tested had results that were at least 5 percent above or below accurate measures. Accurate cholesterol measurement is an absolute necessity for an accurate Reversal Profile.

While you're at it, have your doctor measure your height and weight. Although your home scale is fine for daily monitoring, the one in your doctor's office is usually more accurate and less prone to fluctuation.

Since you are paying for an office visit anyway, ask him for a routine physical examination to see if you can safely start a fitness program. I generally recommend such an examination to people starting an exercise program after the age of thirty-five. Even at that tender age, heart disease has been known to have already crept up on some people, making exercise more dangerous than they may know. Stress tests are also necessary for people with heart disease or those who are coronary-prone.

Although a stress test isn't a necessary gauge of whether or not you can exercise, it might be a useful test to have if you can afford it. It reveals exactly how much oxygen your body consumes per kilogram of body weight, a factor that improves as you lose weight and become more fit. It is one more valuable number in charting your progress on the reversal diet program.

Even if you don't have a stress test (and I consider it optional unless your personal physician insists upon it) there are other ways to chart your improvements through fitness. Keep a record of the number of calories burned in exercise each day and how you feel after doing it. You can also keep a record of your resting pulse rate, although it isn't among the goals of the reversal program. Resting pulse rate is an indicator of improved fitness, since the heart slows down and beats more efficiently when it is fit. You will most likely have a steady drop in resting pulse rate while following a regular exercise program.

The goals for these seven factors are listed in your Reversal Profile along with spaces for you to fill in your own numbers. There are two Reversal Profile diaries, one for you to complete now and one to complete in three months. That way you can see in black and white the changes you have made.

Most people are surprised at how quickly they respond to this program. Generally speaking, they lose weight (which about 26 percent of Americans should do anyway) and feel a substantial increase in their energy levels.

That response is understandable, since one of the real beauties of the reversal diet program is that it gets visible results without being a difficult program to stay on. It gets less obvious results, too, by greatly reducing and oftentimes virtually erasing your risk of heart diseases.

Food Diary Advice

The most time-consuming, yet interesting, part of your reversal profile is the diet diary. Its purpose is to keep track of your daily bread—and the other foods you eat. Since your diet can affect virtually every goal of reversal, it is probably the most important factor in reversing heart disease. After all, diet can change your serum-cholesterol level, LDL cholesterol, and total cholesterol/HDL ratio, your blood pressure and blood-sugar levels, and your body weight.

Rest assured that not everything you eat is wrong. In fact, very little will probably have to be given up on the reversal diet. As a physician who has spent more than forty years helping people make life-style changes, I find this fact to be good news. There is one axiom that holds true when trying to change the way people live: *He who changes least, changes best.* The less drastic changes you have to make in the way you eat, exercise, and react to the world around you, the more likely you are to make those changes a part of your life instead of a passing fancy.

One reason so many life-style change programs fail is that they require you to make extraordinary alterations in living and eating habits. Most people can stay on a "radical change" program for only a short period of time. Then, after a while, as one patient put it, "I begin to feel like I'm living another person's life."

The fact is that these programs usually do make you live someone else's life. Rarely do they help you examine your own life-style habits to see what—if anything—you are doing that might contribute to heart disease. Instead many of them tell you that everything you have done in your life is wrong and that you must make substantial changes to get the desired results.

Thus many people begin with good intentions that erode. They start to cheat, going off their restrictive diets a little bit at a time until they find that they have totally relapsed. Several studies show that from 40 to 60 percent of people who begin a life-style program calling for a radically different diet leave that program within the first year.

Relapse is one of the most frustrating problems of a life-style program for both doctor and patient. But in my own work I have found that a relapse is not inevitable. By first having my patients keep a seven-day diet diary that we can analyze, I have found that most of them need to make very few changes to follow the reversal diet program. For instance, a patient's diet might be well within the reversal range if it weren't for a daily helping of rich ice cream (one of the public enemies of cholesterol control and weight loss) to put her or him over the cholesterol and fat quotient. The key in this case would be to substitute nonfat, no-cholesterol yogurt or one of the appealing recipes in the back of the book. Patients with a fondness for red meat can discover how to trim fat and broil meat, or mix small amounts of it with vegetables so they can still have the benefit of its taste. *He who changes least, changes best.* If you can make small changes without feeling deprived, why do more?

Using the Seven-Day Diary*

We have included two seven-day diaries—one to be completed now and the other, in three months. At the bottom of each page are the reversal goals for diet, exercise, and body weight. When each day's dietary intake and calories burned in exercise are tallied, you can compare the numbers you attained to the reversal numbers next to them and see immediately what changes have to be made. At the end of only seven days you will have an idea of how to bring your diet into the reversal range.

Following the seven-day diary is a worksheet entitled "Taking Stock." The purpose of this worksheet is to keep track of the great "offenders" in your diet, the foods that contribute the greatest number of saturated-fat calories, the greatest amount of cholesterol, or the most sodium. These are the foods you must cut back on or cut out entirely.

How do you find the composition of the foods you eat? At the end of this chapter is a food table, a lengthy list of common foods and their content of total fats, saturated fat, calories, cholesterol, and sodium. This provides the data necessary to determine the composition of your meals.

There are some important things to remember before launching into a personal dietary analysis:

• **Write it all down:** Make sure you write down *everything* you eat. That means individual ingredients, too. When you include a salad, for example, measure the salad dressing and write down the amount and type, the various vegetables, and anything else you might put on it, such as cheese or meat. The same is true of mixed dishes and casseroles. If they aren't listed in the Mixed Dishes section of the food

---

* Reproduced with permission.
© *Dietary Treatment of Hypercholesterolemia, A Manual for Patients*, 1988.
Copyright American Heart Association

table on page 115, you will be able to compile accurately the composition of each dish eaten by listing the ingredients individually.

Also, no amount of food is too small or too low in calories *not* to be included in the diary. Write down every peanut, every chocolate candy, even every apple. Every shred of dietary information is important.

• *Don't change what you eat:* I know how hard it is not to change what you eat when keeping a diary because I have done it myself. The reason for these changes is clear: You begin to gain insight when you watch yourself. You may pick up a handful of peanuts and in counting them realize that at seven calories per peanut, you are holding 140 calories in your hand. Rather than eat them, the temptation might be to put them back.

For this week only, grin and eat them. Changes can come the following week when you begin reaching for your reversal goals.

• *Weigh everything you eat:* For the week of this diary, weigh everything you eat, if possible. Although the food table lists a weight for each food that approximates a normal portion, weighing everything lets you see if what you are eating is equal to the amount expressed in the table. If weighing is not practical, at least estimate the weight of the portion.

Weighing food in restaurants is not usually the socially acceptable thing to do. Instead of producing a scale and weighing your meal, ask the chef to provide the information. For information on fast foods, see the Fast Foods section in this chapter's food table.

• *Keep track of calories burned each day:* The number of calories you burn each day vary according to height, weight, age, metabolism, and the amount of exercise you do. An active man burns about fifteen calories per pound each day, which means a man weighing 180 pounds would burn about 2,700 calories a day. An inactive man, on the other hand, burns about thirteen calories per pound each day, which means he uses about 2,350 calories each day.

To estimate roughly the number of calories you need to *maintain* and to *attain* your desired weight,* complete the following equation:

---

* Your desired or ideal body weight also can be estimated from the height, weight, and body frame chart on page 54, or from a weight recommended by your physician. Incidentally, many people find that their ideal body weight was the same as their weight at the age of twenty-five years. This equation tells you how many calories you need to maintain your current weight or to attain your ideal weight.

Body Weight (lbs)		Calories per pound		Calories per day
Active Man				
Present _____	×	15	=	_____
Desired _____	×	15	=	_____
Inactive Man				
Present _____	×	13	=	_____
Desired _____	×	13	=	_____
Active Woman				
Present _____	×	12	=	_____
Desired _____	×	12	=	_____
Inactive Woman				
Present _____	×	10	=	_____
Desired _____	×	10	=	_____

First See Your Physician

Ready to begin? First consult your physician about your plan to partic-ipate in the Reversal Diet Program. Let your spouse and closest friends know that their help and approval are necessary for your success. Get a physical examination from your physician, including the blood tests, blood pressure readings, electrocardiogram, exercise test, and mea-surement of body weight and height needed to complete your Reversal Profile.

If you are slightly overweight—say 5 to 10 pounds—you can prob-ably lose that weight on your own. One recommendation would be to find your ideal weight, however derived, and eat no more than it takes to attain and maintain that weight. For instance, if you weigh 170 pounds, but should weigh 160 pounds, eat just enough calories to "feed" that ideal weight and let the ten extra pounds shrivel away, at the rate of 1 to 2 pounds each week. If you are more than 10 to 20 pounds overweight, or lack willpower, consult your physician for a sensible weight-loss program, and the necessary psychological support to help you change your eating habits.

Permanent weight loss isn't easy, as many people can attest. For every pound of excess body weight, you are carrying 3,500 extra cal-ories. For example, if you are 20 pounds over ideal weight, you are carrying 70,000 *extra* calories. To reach your Reversal Goal, you have the option of getting rid of these extra calories by restricting the amount of food you eat, or by increasing the amount of exercise, or by a combination of the two. Weight loss is accomplished more favorably (more fat and less muscle loss) by the combination.

To lose this or greater amounts of body fat sensibly, the help of your physician is essential.

The two of you should also agree upon the type and amount of exercise you should do for this program.

Remember: *Your reversal goals must be realistic and acceptable to you and your physician.*

There is probably no better weight loss method than the Reversal Diet Program, which combines diet and exercise. Not only is it a realistic regimen to stay on, but the low-fat/high-fiber foods recommended make it possible to eat until you feel full and still lose weight.

Ready? Begin with The Reversal Profile.

THE REVERSAL PROFILE

_____

Name

_____

Date

This is the beginning of your reversal diet program. Go to your doctor for the necessary blood tests that will determine your current total serum cholesterol, your total cholesterol/HDL ratio, and your blood-sugar level. Also, have your doctor weigh you and take your blood pressure.

Record all the numbers for each of these tests on the next page.

For the next week, record your diet and exercise habits in the diet and exercise diary. Use the food table on pages 108–126 to figure the breakdown of your daily consumption of food. Try not to change what you eat or how much you exercise, since you are trying to obtain a true record of your habits. Honesty is the best policy.

The time to make changes is at the end of the week when you have an exact understanding of your eating and exercise patterns.

Another Reversal Profile and Diet/Exercise Diary follows this one.

It is to be filled out in three months to see how well you have made the changes detailed in Chapters 4 through 8.

REVERSAL GOALS AND YOUR PROFILE

Reversal Goal for Cholesterol: Total Serum Cholesterol under 200 mg/dl

• Your current serum cholesterol: _____ mg/dl

Reversal Goal for Total Cholesterol/HDL Cholesterol Ratio: 3.5 (total) to 1 (HDL)

• Current total cholesterol/HDL ratio: _____ to 1

Reversal Goal for Blood Pressure: 140/90 or less

• Current blood pressure reading: _____

Reversal Goal for Body Weight: Fill in weight based on height/ weight from chart on page 54

• Current body weight: _____ pounds

Reversal Goal for Blood-Sugar Level: 80 to 105 mg/dl

• Current blood-sugar level: _____

Reversal Goal for Calories Expended in Exercise: 150 to 300 Calories per Day, 1,050 to 2,000 per Week

• Current calories burned weekly in exercise (calculate by totaling daily exercise from the seven-day diary): _____

Reversal Goal for Daily Caloric Intake: Personal physician's recommendation or your own estimate from applying ideal body weight to equation on page 71: _____

• Current daily caloric intake (averaged from the seven-day diary): _____

Reversal Goal for Tobacco Use: Zero Tobacco in Any Form

• Current tobacco use: _____

DIET/EXERCISE DIARY—DAY 1

Food and Method of Preparation	Amount (g)	Total Calories	Fat (cals)	Sat. Fat (cals)	Choles. (mg)	Sodium (mg)
1						
2						
3						
4						
5						
6						
7						
8						
9						
10						
11						
12						
13						
14						
15						
16						
17						
18						
19						
20						
21						
22						
23						
24						
25						

Food and Method of Preparation	Amount (g)	Total Calories	Fat (cals)	Sat. Fat (cals)	Choles. (mg)	Sodium (mg)
26						
27						
28						
29						
30						
31						
32						
33						
34						
35						
36						
37						
38						

Totals: _____

	Calories	Fat (cals)	Sat. Fat (cals)	Choles. (mg)	Sodium (mg)

* To figure % fat cals: _____ ÷ _____ × 100 = _____

    Equation: (fat cals) ÷ (total cals) × 100 = total fat cals

* To figure % sat. fat cals:_____ ÷ _____ × 100 = _____

    Equation: (sat. fat cals) ÷ (total cals) × 100 = sat. fat cals

Exercise Record (calories burned in all exercise today, including walking, stair climbing, etc. For Calorie Chart, see Table 12)

Type: _____ cals burned _____ Type: _____ cals burned _____

Type: _____ cals burned _____ Type: _____ cals burned _____

Total calories burned in exercise: _____

Reversal goals:
Total cals = _____ (from Reversal Profile)
Fat = 30% total calories
Saturated fat = 10% total calories—or less
Cholesterol = 300 mg or less per day
Sodium = 1,100–3,300 mg or less per day
Exercise = 150–300 cals per day
Weight goal _____ lbs (from Table 3)

Levels attained today:
Total cals = _____
% Fat cals = _____
% Sat. fat cals = _____
Cholesterol = _____ mg
Sodium = _____ mg
Exercise cals _____
Morning weight _____ lbs

DIET/EXERCISE DIARY—DAY 2

Food and Method of Preparation	Amount (g)	Total Calories	Fat (cals)	Sat. Fat (cals)	Choles. (mg)	Sodium (mg)
1						
2						
3						
4						
5						
6						
7						
8						
9						
10						
11						
12						
13						
14						
15						
16						
17						
18						
19						
20						
21						
22						
23						
24						
25						

Food and Method of Preparation	Amount (g)	Total Calories	Fat (cals)	Sat. Fat (cals)	Choles. (mg)	Sodium (mg)
26						
27						
28						
29						
30						
31						
32						
33						
34						
35						
36						
37						
38						

Totals: _____

	Calories	Fat (cals)	Sat. Fat (cals)	Choles. (mg)	Sodium (mg)

* To figure % fat cals: _____ ÷ _____ × 100 = _____
  Equation: (fat cals) ÷ (total cals) × 100 = total fat cals
* To figure % sat. fat cals:_____ ÷ _____ × 100 = _____
  Equation: (sat. fat cals) ÷ (total cals) × 100 = sat. fat cals

Exercise Record (calories burned in all exercise today, including walking, stair climbing, etc. For Calorie Chart, see Table 12)
Type: _____ cals burned _____ Type: _____ cals burned _____
Type: _____ cals burned _____ Type: _____ cals burned _____
Total calories burned in exercise: _____

Reversal goals:
Total cals = _____ (from Reversal Profile)
Fat = 30% total calories
Saturated fat = 10% total calories—or less
Cholesterol = 300 mg or less per day
Sodium = 1,100–3,300 mg or less per day
Exercise = 150–300 cals per day
Weight goal _____ lbs (from Table 3)

Levels attained today:
Total cals = _____
% Fat cals = _____
% Sat. fat cals = _____
Cholesterol = _____ mg
Sodium = _____ mg
Exercise cals _____
Morning weight _____ lbs

DIET/EXERCISE DIARY—DAY 3

Food and Method of Preparation	Amount (g)	Total Calories	Fat (cals)	Sat. Fat (cals)	Choles. (mg)	Sodium (mg)
1						
2						
3						
4						
5						
6						
7						
8						
9						
10						
11						
12						
13						
14						
15						
16						
17						
18						
19						
20						
21						
22						
23						
24						
25						

Food and Method of Preparation	Amount (g)	Total Calories	Fat (cals)	Sat. Fat (cals)	Choles. (mg)	Sodium (mg)
26						
27						
28						
29						
30						
31						
32						
33						
34						
35						
36						
37						
38						

Totals: _____

	Calories	Fat (cals)	Sat. Fat (cals)	Choles. (mg)	Sodium (mg)

* To figure % fat cals: _____ ÷ _____ × 100 = _____
  Equation: (fat cals) ÷ (total cals) × 100 = total fat cals
* To figure % sat. fat cals:_____ ÷ _____ × 100 = _____
  Equation: (sat. fat cals) ÷ (total cals) × 100 = sat. fat cals

Exercise Record (calories burned in all exercise today, including walking, stair climbing, etc. For Calorie Chart, see Table 12)
Type: _____ cals burned _____ Type: _____ cals burned _____
Type: _____ cals burned _____ Type: _____ cals burned _____
Total calories burned in exercise: _____

Reversal goals:
Total cals = _____ (from Reversal Profile)
Fat = 30% total calories
Saturated fat = 10% total calories—or less
Cholesterol = 300 mg or less per day
Sodium = 1,100–3,300 mg or less per day
Exercise = 150–300 cals per day
Weight goal _____ lbs (from Table 3)

Levels attained today:
Total cals = _____
% Fat cals = _____
% Sat. fat cals = _____
Cholesterol = _____ mg
Sodium = _____ mg
Exercise cals _____
Morning weight _____ lbs

DIET/EXERCISE DIARY—DAY 4

Food and Method of Preparation	Amount (g)	Total Calories	Fat (cals)	Sat. Fat (cals)	Choles. (mg)	Sodium (mg)
1						
2						
3						
4						
5						
6						
7						
8						
9						
10						
11						
12						
13						
14						
15						
16						
17						
18						
19						
20						
21						
22						
23						
24						
25						

Food and Method of Preparation	Amount (g)	Total Calories	Fat (cals)	Sat. Fat (cals)	Choles. (mg)	Sodium (mg)
26						
27						
28						
29						
30						
31						
32						
33						
34						
35						
36						
37						
38						

Totals: _____

	Calories	Fat (cals)	Sat. Fat (cals)	Choles. (mg)	Sodium (mg)

* To figure % fat cals: _____ ÷ _____ × 100 = _____
  Equation: (fat cals) ÷ (total cals) × 100 = total fat cals
* To figure % sat. fat cals: _____ ÷ _____ × 100 = _____
  Equation: (sat. fat cals) ÷ (total cals) × 100 = sat. fat cals

Exercise Record (calories burned in all exercise today, including walking, stair climbing, etc. For Calorie Chart, see Table 12)
Type: _____ cals burned _____ Type: _____ cals burned _____
Type: _____ cals burned _____ Type: _____ cals burned _____
Total calories burned in exercise: _____

Reversal goals:
Total cals = _____ (from Reversal Profile)
Fat = 30% total calories
Saturated fat = 10% total calories—or less
Cholesterol = 300 mg or less per day
Sodium = 1,100–3,300 mg or less per day
Exercise = 150–300 cals per day
Weight goal _____ lbs (from Table 3)

Levels attained today:
Total cals = _____
% Fat cals = _____
% Sat. fat cals = _____
Cholesterol = _____ mg
Sodium = _____ mg
Exercise cals _____
Morning weight _____ lbs

DIET/EXERCISE DIARY—DAY 5

Food and Method of Preparation	Amount (g)	Total Calories	Fat (cals)	Sat. Fat (cals)	Choles. (mg)	Sodium (mg)
1						
2						
3						
4						
5						
6						
7						
8						
9						
10						
11						
12						
13						
14						
15						
16						
17						
18						
19						
20						
21						
22						
23						
24						
25						

Food and Method of Preparation	Amount (g)	Total Calories	Fat (cals)	Sat. Fat (cals)	Choles. (mg)	Sodium (mg)
26						
27						
28						
29						
30						
31						
32						
33						
34						
35						
36						
37						
38						

Totals: _____

	Calories	Fat (cals)	Sat. Fat (cals)	Choles. (mg)	Sodium (mg)

* To figure % fat cals: _____ ÷ _____ × 100 = _____
  Equation:　　(fat cals) ÷ (total cals) × 100 = total fat cals

* To figure % sat. fat cals: _____ ÷ _____ × 100 = _____
  Equation:　　(sat. fat cals) ÷ (total cals) × 100 = sat. fat cals

Exercise Record (calories burned in all exercise today, including walking, stair climbing, etc. For Calorie Chart, see Table 12)

Type: _____ cals burned _____　Type: _____ cals burned _____
Type: _____ cals burned _____　Type: _____ cals burned _____
Total calories burned in exercise: _____

Reversal goals:
Total cals = _____ (from Reversal Profile)
Fat = 30% total calories
Saturated fat = 10% total calories—or less
Cholesterol = 300 mg or less per day
Sodium = 1,100–3,300 mg or less per day
Exercise = 150–300 cals per day
Weight goal _____ lbs (from Table 3)

Levels attained today:
Total cals = _____
% Fat cals = _____
% Sat. fat cals = _____
Cholesterol = _____ mg
Sodium = _____ mg
Exercise cals _____
Morning weight _____ lbs

DIET/EXERCISE DIARY—DAY 6

Food and Method of Preparation	Amount (g)	Total Calories	Fat (cals)	Sat. Fat (cals)	Choles. (mg)	Sodium (mg)
1						
2						
3						
4						
5						
6						
7						
8						
9						
10						
11						
12						
13						
14						
15						
16						
17						
18						
19						
20						
21						
22						
23						
24						
25						

Food and Method of Preparation	Amount (g)	Total Calories	Fat (cals)	Sat. Fat (cals)	Choles. (mg)	Sodium (mg)
26						
27						
28						
29						
30						
31						
32						
33						
34						
35						
36						
37						
38						

Totals: _____

	Calories	Fat (cals)	Sat. Fat (cals)	Choles. (mg)	Sodium (mg)

* To figure % fat cals: _____ ÷ _____ × 100 = _____

  Equation: (fat cals) ÷ (total cals) × 100 = total fat cals

* To figure % sat. fat cals: _____ ÷ _____ × 100 = _____

  Equation: (sat. fat cals) ÷ (total cals) × 100 = sat. fat cals

Exercise Record (calories burned in all exercise today, including walking, stair climbing, etc. For Calorie Chart, see Table 12)

Type: _____ cals burned _____   Type: _____ cals burned _____

Type: _____ cals burned _____   Type: _____ cals burned _____

Total calories burned in exercise: _____

Reversal goals:

Total cals = _____ (from Reversal Profile)

Fat = 30% total calories

Saturated fat = 10% total calories—or less

Cholesterol = 300 mg or less per day

Sodium = 1,100–3,300 mg or less per day

Exercise = 150–300 cals per day

Weight goal _____ lbs (from Table 3)

Levels attained today:

Total cals = _____

% Fat cals = _____

% Sat. fat cals = _____

Cholesterol = _____ mg

Sodium = _____ mg

Exercise cals _____

Morning weight _____ lbs

DIET/EXERCISE DIARY—DAY 7

Food and Method of Preparation	Amount (g)	Total Calories	Fat (cals)	Sat. Fat (cals)	Choles. (mg)	Sodium (mg)
1						
2						
3						
4						
5						
6						
7						
8						
9						
10						
11						
12						
13						
14						
15						
16						
17						
18						
19						
20						
21						
22						
23						
24						
25						

Food and Method of Preparation	Amount (g)	Total Calories	Fat (cals)	Sat. Fat (cals)	Choles. (mg)	Sodium (mg)
26						
27						
28						
29						
30						
31						
32						
33						
34						
35						
36						
37						
38						

Totals: _____

	Calories	Fat (cals)	Sat. Fat (cals)	Choles. (mg)	Sodium (mg)

* To figure % fat cals: _____ ÷ _____ × 100 = _____

   Equation: (fat cals) ÷ (total cals) × 100 = total fat cals

* To figure % sat. fat cals:_____ ÷ _____ × 100 = _____

   Equation: (sat. fat cals) ÷ (total cals) × 100 = sat. fat cals

Exercise Record (calories burned in all exercise today, including walking, stair climbing, etc. For Calorie Chart, see Table 12)

Type: _____ cals burned _____ Type: _____ cals burned _____
Type: _____ cals burned _____ Type: _____ cals burned _____
Total calories burned in exercise: _____

Reversal goals:
Total cals = _____ (from Reversal Profile)
Fat = 30% total calories
Saturated fat = 10% total calories—or less
Cholesterol = 300 mg or less per day
Sodium = 1,100–3,300 mg or less per day
Exercise = 150–300 cals per day
Weight goal _____ lbs (from Table 3)

Levels attained today:
Total cals = _____
% Fat cals = _____
% Sat. fat cals = _____
Cholesterol = _____ mg
Sodium = _____ mg
Exercise cals _____
Morning weight _____ lbs

TAKING STOCK

Review the diary of the past week and identify the Great Offenders—foods high in cholesterol, fats, and sodium that you could eat less of or omit entirely.

Food and Method of Preparation	Amount (g)	Total Calories	Fat (cals)	Sat. Fat (cals)	Choles. (mg)	Sodium (mg)
1						
2						
3						
4						
5						
6						
7						
8						
9						
10						
11						
12						
13						
14						
15						
16						
17						
18						
19						
20						
21						
22						
23						
24						

Great Offender Substitutes
(Foods lower in cholesterol, fats, and sodium that can replace the Great Offenders can be found in Chapters 4 and 11.)

Food and Method of Preparation	Amount (g)	Total Calories	Fat (cals)	Sat. Fat (cals)	Choles. (mg)	Sodium (mg)
1						
2						
3						
4						
5						
6						
7						
8						
9						
10						
11						
12						
13						
14						
15						
16						
17						
18						
19						
20						
21						
22						
23						
24						

REVERSAL PROFILE THREE-MONTH PROGRESS REPORT

_____

Name

_____

Date

This is your three-month reversal diet progress report. By now you should have read the book and made the recommended life-style changes. The progress report will show you how much closer you are to meeting the goals of the reversal program.

Once again, go to your doctor for the necessary blood tests that determine your current total serum cholesterol, your total cholesterol/ HDL ratio, and your blood-sugar level. Also, have your doctor weigh you and take your blood pressure.

Record all the numbers for each of these tests on the next page.

The next week, record your diet and exercise habits in the diet and exercise diary. Try not to change what you eat or how much you exercise, since you are trying to obtain a true record of your habits.

Compare the results in this profile to the Reversal Goals and the results of your first profile. Depending upon the changes that were needed, your numbers should be substantially improved if not well within the reversal goals.

REVERSAL GOALS AND YOUR THREE-MONTH PROFILE

Reversal Goal for Cholesterol: Total Serum Cholesterol under 200 mg/dl

- Your current serum cholesterol: _____ mg/dl

Reversal Goal for Total Cholesterol/HDL Cholesterol Ratio: 3.5 (total) to 1 (HDL)

- Current total cholesterol/HDL ratio: _____ to 1

Reversal Goal for Blood Pressure: 140/90 or less

- Current blood pressure reading: _____

Reversal Goal for Body Weight: Fill in weight based on height/weight from chart on page 54

- Current body weight: _____ pounds

Reversal Goal for Blood-Sugar Level: 80 to 105 mg/dl

- Current blood-sugar level: _____

Reversal Goal for Calories Expended in Exercise: 150 to 300 Calories per Day, 1,050 to 2,000 per Week

- Current calories burned weekly in exercise (calculate by totaling daily exercise from the seven-day diary): _____

Reversal Goal for Daily Caloric Intake: Personal physician's recommendation or your own estimate from applying ideal body weight to equation on page 71: _____

- Current daily caloric intake (averaged from the seven-day diary): _____

Reversal Goal for Tobacco Use: Zero Tobacco in Any Form

- Current tobacco use: _____

DIET/EXERCISE DIARY—DAY 1

Food and Method of Preparation	Amount (g)	Total Calories	Fat (cals)	Sat. Fat (cals)	Choles. (mg)	Sodium (mg)
1						
2						
3						
4						
5						
6						
7						
8						
9						
10						
11						
12						
13						
14						
15						
16						
17						
18						
19						
20						
21						
22						
23						
24						
25						

Food and Method of Preparation	Amount (g)	Total Calories	Fat (cals)	Sat. Fat (cals)	Choles. (mg)	Sodium (mg)
26						
27						
28						
29						
30						
31						
32						
33						
34						
35						
36						
37						
38						

Totals: _____

	Calories	Fat (cals)	Sat. Fat (cals)	Choles. (mg)	Sodium (mg)

* To figure % fat cals: _____ ÷ _____ × 100 = _____
  Equation: (fat cals) ÷ (total cals) × 100 = total fat cals

* To figure % sat. fat cals: _____ ÷ _____ × 100 = _____
  Equation: (sat. fat cals) ÷ (total cals) × 100 = sat. fat cals

Exercise Record (calories burned in all exercise today, including walking, stair climbing, etc. For Calorie Chart, see Table 12)

Type: _____ cals burned _____ Type: _____ cals burned _____
Type: _____ cals burned _____ Type: _____ cals burned _____
Total calories burned in exercise: _____

Reversal goals:
Total cals = _____ (from Reversal Profile)
Fat = 30% total calories
Saturated fat = 10% total calories—or less
Cholesterol = 300 mg or less per day
Sodium = 1,100–3,300 mg or less per day
Exercise = 150–300 cals per day
Weight goal _____ lbs (from Table 3)

Levels attained today:
Total cals = _____
% Fat cals = _____
% Sat. fat cals = _____
Cholesterol = _____ mg
Sodium = _____ mg
Exercise cals _____
Morning weight _____ lbs

DIET/EXERCISE DIARY—DAY 2

Food and Method of Preparation	Amount (g)	Total Calories	Fat (cals)	Sat. Fat (cals)	Choles. (mg)	Sodium (mg)
1						
2						
3						
4						
5						
6						
7						
8						
9						
10						
11						
12						
13						
14						
15						
16						
17						
18						
19						
20						
21						
22						
23						
24						
25						

Food and Method of Preparation	Amount (g)	Total Calories	Fat (cals)	Sat. Fat (cals)	Choles. (mg)	Sodium (mg)
26						
27						
28						
29						
30						
31						
32						
33						
34						
35						
36						
37						
38						

Totals: _____

	Calories	Fat (cals)	Sat. Fat (cals)	Choles. (mg)	Sodium (mg)

* To figure % fat cals: _____ ÷ _____ × 100 = _____
    Equation: (fat cals) ÷ (total cals) × 100 = total fat cals

* To figure % sat. fat cals:_____ ÷ _____ × 100 = _____
    Equation: (sat. fat cals) ÷ (total cals) × 100 = sat. fat cals

Exercise Record (calories burned in all exercise today, including walking, stair climbing, etc. For Calorie Chart, see Table 12)

Type: _____ cals burned _____   Type: _____ cals burned _____
Type: _____ cals burned _____   Type: _____ cals burned _____
Total calories burned in exercise: _____

Reversal goals:
Total cals = _____ (from Reversal Profile)
Fat = 30% total calories
Saturated fat = 10% total calories—or less
Cholesterol = 300 mg or less per day
Sodium = 1,100–3,300 mg or less per day
Exercise = 150–300 cals per day
Weight goal _____ lbs (from Table 3)

Levels attained today:
Total cals = _____
% Fat cals = _____
% Sat. fat cals = _____
Cholesterol = _____ mg
Sodium = _____ mg
Exercise cals _____
Morning weight _____ lbs

DIET/EXERCISE DIARY—DAY 3

Food and Method of Preparation	Amount (g)	Total Calories	Fat (cals)	Sat. Fat (cals)	Choles. (mg)	Sodium (mg)
1						
2						
3						
4						
5						
6						
7						
8						
9						
10						
11						
12						
13						
14						
15						
16						
17						
18						
19						
20						
21						
22						
23						
24						
25						

Food and Method of Preparation	Amount (g)	Total Calories	Fat (cals)	Sat. Fat (cals)	Choles. (mg)	Sodium (mg)
26						
27						
28						
29						
30						
31						
32						
33						
34						
35						
36						
37						
38						

Totals: _____

	Calories	Fat (cals)	Sat. Fat (cals)	Choles. (mg)	Sodium (mg)

* To figure % fat cals: _____ ÷ _____ × 100 = _____
    Equation: (fat cals) ÷ (total cals) × 100 = total fat cals

* To figure % sat. fat cals:_____ ÷ _____ × 100 = _____
    Equation: (sat. fat cals) ÷ (total cals) × 100 = sat. fat cals

Exercise Record (calories burned in all exercise today, including walking, stair climbing, etc. For Calorie Chart, see Table 12)
Type: _____ cals burned _____ Type: _____ cals burned _____
Type: _____ cals burned _____ Type: _____ cals burned _____
Total calories burned in exercise: _____

Reversal goals:
Total cals = _____ (from Reversal Profile)
Fat = 30% total calories
Saturated fat = 10% total calories—or less
Cholesterol = 300 mg or less per day
Sodium = 1,100–3,300 mg or less per day
Exercise = 150–300 cals per day
Weight goal _____ lbs (from Table 3)

Levels attained today:
Total cals = _____
% Fat cals = _____
% Sat. fat cals = _____
Cholesterol = _____ mg
Sodium = _____ mg
Exercise cals _____
Morning weight _____ lbs

DIET/EXERCISE DIARY—DAY 4

Food and Method of Preparation	Amount (g)	Total Calories	Fat (cals)	Sat. Fat (cals)	Choles. (mg)	Sodium (mg)
1						
2						
3						
4						
5						
6						
7						
8						
9						
10						
11						
12						
13						
14						
15						
16						
17						
18						
19						
20						
21						
22						
23						
24						
25						

Food and Method of Preparation	Amount (g)	Total Calories	Fat (cals)	Sat. Fat (cals)	Choles. (mg)	Sodium (mg)
26						
27						
28						
29						
30						
31						
32						
33						
34						
35						
36						
37						
38						

Totals: _____

	Calories	Fat (cals)	Sat. Fat (cals)	Choles. (mg)	Sodium (mg)

* To figure % fat cals: _____ ÷ _____ × 100 = _____
   Equation: (fat cals) ÷ (total cals) × 100 = total fat cals

* To figure % sat. fat cals:_____ ÷ _____ × 100 = _____
   Equation: (sat. fat cals) ÷ (total cals) × 100 = sat. fat cals

Exercise Record (calories burned in all exercise today, including walking, stair climbing, etc. For Calorie Chart, see Table 12)

Type: _____ cals burned _____   Type: _____ cals burned _____
Type: _____ cals burned _____   Type: _____ cals burned _____
Total calories burned in exercise: _____

Reversal goals:
Total cals = _____ (from Reversal Profile)
Fat = 30% total calories
Saturated fat = 10% total calories—or less
Cholesterol = 300 mg or less per day
Sodium = 1,100–3,300 mg or less per day
Exercise = 150–300 cals per day
Weight goal _____ lbs (from Table 3)

Levels attained today:
Total cals = _____
% Fat cals = _____
% Sat. fat cals = _____
Cholesterol = _____ mg
Sodium = _____ mg
Exercise cals _____
Morning weight _____ lbs

DIET/EXERCISE DIARY—DAY 5

Food and Method of Preparation	Amount (g)	Total Calories	Fat (cals)	Sat. Fat (cals)	Choles. (mg)	Sodium (mg)
1						
2						
3						
4						
5						
6						
7						
8						
9						
10						
11						
12						
13						
14						
15						
16						
17						
18						
19						
20						
21						
22						
23						
24						
25						

Food and Method of Preparation	Amount (g)	Total Calories	Fat (cals)	Sat. Fat (cals)	Choles. (mg)	Sodium (mg)
26						
27						
28						
29						
30						
31						
32						
33						
34						
35						
36						
37						
38						

Totals: _____

	Calories	Fat (cals)	Sat. Fat (cals)	Choles. (mg)	Sodium (mg)

* To figure % fat cals: _____ ÷ _____ × 100 = _____

    Equation: (fat cals) ÷ (total cals) × 100 = total fat cals

* To figure % sat. fat cals: _____ ÷ _____ × 100 = _____

    Equation: (sat. fat cals) ÷ (total cals) × 100 = sat. fat cals

Exercise Record (calories burned in all exercise today, including walking, stair climbing, etc. For Calorie Chart, see Table 12)

Type: _____ cals burned _____   Type: _____ cals burned _____

Type: _____ cals burned _____   Type: _____ cals burned _____

Total calories burned in exercise: _____

Reversal goals:
Total cals = _____ (from Reversal Profile)
Fat = 30% total calories
Saturated fat = 10% total calories—or less
Cholesterol = 300 mg or less per day
Sodium = 1,100–3,300 mg or less per day
Exercise = 150–300 cals per day
Weight goal _____ lbs (from Table 3)

Levels attained today:
Total cals = _____
% Fat cals = _____
% Sat. fat cals = _____
Cholesterol = _____ mg
Sodium = _____ mg
Exercise cals _____
Morning weight _____ lbs

DIET/EXERCISE DIARY—DAY 6

Food and Method of Preparation	Amount (g)	Total Calories	Fat (cals)	Sat. Fat (cals)	Choles. (mg)	Sodium (mg)
1						
2						
3						
4						
5						
6						
7						
8						
9						
10						
11						
12						
13						
14						
15						
16						
17						
18						
19						
20						
21						
22						
23						
24						
25						

Food and Method of Preparation	Amount (g)	Total Calories	Fat (cals)	Sat. Fat (cals)	Choles. (mg)	Sodium (mg)
26						
27						
28						
29						
30						
31						
32						
33						
34						
35						
36						
37						
38						

Totals: _____

	Calories	Fat (cals)	Sat. Fat (cals)	Choles. (mg)	Sodium (mg)

* To figure % fat cals: _____ ÷ _____ × 100 = _____

    Equation: (fat cals) ÷ (total cals) × 100 = total fat cals

* To figure % sat. fat cals: _____ ÷ _____ × 100 = _____

    Equation: (sat. fat cals) ÷ (total cals) × 100 = sat. fat cals

Exercise Record (calories burned in all exercise today, including walking, stair climbing, etc. For Calorie Chart, see Table 12)

Type: _____ cals burned _____ Type: _____ cals burned _____

Type: _____ cals burned _____ Type: _____ cals burned _____

Total calories burned in exercise: _____

Reversal goals:
Total cals = _____ (from Reversal Profile)
Fat = 30% total calories
Saturated fat = 10% total calories—or less
Cholesterol = 300 mg or less per day
Sodium = 1,100–3,300 mg or less per day
Exercise = 150–300 cals per day
Weight goal _____ lbs (from Table 3)

Levels attained today:
Total cals = _____
% Fat cals = _____
% Sat. fat cals = _____
Cholesterol = _____ mg
Sodium = _____ mg
Exercise cals _____
Morning weight _____ lbs

DIET/EXERCISE DIARY—DAY 7

Food and Method of Preparation	Amount (g)	Total Calories	Fat (cals)	Sat. Fat (cals)	Choles. (mg)	Sodium (mg)
1						
2						
3						
4						
5						
6						
7						
8						
9						
10						
11						
12						
13						
14						
15						
16						
17						
18						
19						
20						
21						
22						
23						
24						
25						

Food and Method of Preparation	Amount (g)	Total Calories	Fat (cals)	Sat. Fat (cals)	Choles. (mg)	Sodium (mg)
26						
27						
28						
29						
30						
31						
32						
33						
34						
35						
36						
37						
38						

Totals: _____

	Calories	Fat (cals)	Sat. Fat (cals)	Choles. (mg)	Sodium (mg)

* To figure % fat cals: _____ ÷ _____ × 100 = _____

Equation: (fat cals) ÷ (total cals) × 100 = total fat cals

* To figure % sat. fat cals: _____ ÷ _____ × 100 = _____

Equation: (sat. fat cals) ÷ (total cals) × 100 = sat. fat cals

Exercise Record (calories burned in all exercise today, including walking, stair climbing, etc. For Calorie Chart, see Table 12)

Type: _____ cals burned _____   Type: _____ cals burned _____
Type: _____ cals burned _____   Type: _____ cals burned _____
Total calories burned in exercise: _____

Reversal goals:
Total cals = _____ (from Reversal Profile)
Fat = 30% total calories
Saturated fat = 10% total calories—or less
Cholesterol = 300 mg or less per day
Sodium = 1,100–3,300 mg or less per day
Exercise = 150–300 cals per day
Weight goal _____ lbs (from Table 3)

Levels attained today:
Total cals = _____
% Fat cals = _____
% Sat. fat cals = _____
Cholesterol = _____ mg
Sodium = _____ mg
Exercise cals _____
Morning weight _____ lbs

TAKING STOCK

Review the diary of the past week and identify the Great Offenders—foods high in cholesterol, fats, and sodium that you could eat less of or omit entirely.

Food and Method of Preparation	Amount (g)	Total Calories	Fat (cals)	Sat. Fat (cals)	Choles. (mg)	Sodium (mg)
1						
2						
3						
4						
5						
6						
7						
8						
9						
10						
11						
12						
13						
14						
15						
16						
17						
18						
19						
20						
21						
22						
23						
24						

Great Offender Substitutes
(Foods lower in cholesterol, fats, and sodium that can replace the Great Offenders
can be found in Chapters 4 and 11.)

Food and Method of Preparation	Amount (g)	Total Calories	Fat (cals)	Sat. Fat (cals)	Choles. (mg)	Sodium (mg)
1						
2						
3						
4						
5						
6						
7						
8						
9						
10						
11						
12						
13						
14						
15						
16						
17						
18						
19						
20						
21						
22						
23						
24						

Table 4.   FOOD TABLE

This table offers analysis of a wide variety of food that comprises the average American diet. Use this table in conjunction with the completed food diaries on the preceding pages to compute your diet profile. Foods are organized under major headings to make it easy to find what you are looking for.

This table has been compiled by the American Heart Association from the United States Department of Agriculture's handbooks on the nutritive value of American foods. It contains most of the foods—or reasonable facsimiles—to closely estimate the content of your daily diet.

SAUCES AND GRAVIES

Dehydrated Sauces   125

Ready-to-Serve Sauces   126

Canned Gravy   126

Dehydrated Gravy   126

ABOUT THE FOOD TABLE

A dash (—) means that a value could not be found, although there is reason to believe that a measurable amount of the nutrient may be present.

ABBREVIATIONS USED IN THE TABLE:

cals	*calories*
Choles.	*cholesterol*
g	*grams*
mg	*milligrams*
Na	*sodium*
oz	*ounces*
Sat. Fatty Acids	*saturated fatty acids*
tr	*trace*

Note: Values have been rounded off; 0.5 or greater is rounded up; 0.4 or less is rounded down.

	Weight (g)	Fat (cals)	Sat. Fatty Acids (cals)	Total (cals)	Choles. (mg)	Na (mg)
MEAT, POULTRY, AND SEAFOOD						
FINFISH						
Catfish, breaded and fried (1 oz)	28	34	8	65	23	79
Cod, Atlantic, cooked, dry heat (1 oz)	28	2	1	30	16	22
Eel, cooked, dry heat (1 oz)	28	38	8	67	46	18
Fish sticks and portions, frozen and reheated (1 oz)	28	31	8	76	31	163
Flounder, cooked, dry heat (1 oz)	28	4	1	33	19	30
Grouper, cooked, dry heat (1 oz)	28	4	1	33	13	15
Haddock, cooked, dry heat (1 oz)	28	3	1	32	21	25
Halibut, cooked, dry heat (1 oz)	28	7	1	40	12	20
Herring, pickled (1 oz)	28	46	6	74	4	247
Mackerel, canned, drained solids (1 oz)	28	16	5	44	22	107
Mackerel, cooked, dry heat (1 oz)	28	45	11	74	21	24
Ocean Perch, cooked, dry heat (1 oz)	28	5	1	34	15	27
Perch, cooked, dry heat (1 oz)	28	3	1	33	33	22
Pike, Northern, cooked, dry heat (1 oz)	28	3	tr	32	14	14

	Weight (g)	Fat (cals)	Sat. Fatty Acids (cals)	Total (cals)	Choles. (mg)	Na (mg)
Finfish *cont.*						
Pollack, Walleye, cooked, dry heat (1 oz)	28	3	1	32	27	33
Pompano, cooked, dry heat (1 oz)	28	31	12	60	18	22
Redfish (see Ocean Perch)						
Rockfish, cooked, dry heat (1 oz)	28	5	1	34	13	22
Salmon, Chinook, smoked (1 oz)	28	11	3	33	7	220 *
Salmon, Chum, canned, drained solids with bone (1 oz)	28	14	4	40	11	138 **
Salmon, Coho, cooked, moist heat (1 oz)	28	19	4	52	14	17
Salmon, Sockeye, canned, drained solids with bone (1 oz)	28	19	5	43	12	153 **
Sardine, Atlantic, canned in oil, drained solids with bone (1 oz)	28	29	tr	59	40	143
Sardine, Pacific, canned in tomato sauce, drained solids with bone (1 oz)	28	31	8	50	17	117
Sea Bass, cooked, dry heat (1 oz)	28	6	2	35	15	25
Scrod (see Cod, Atlantic)						
Snapper, cooked, dry heat (1 oz)	28	5	1	36	13	16
Sole (see Flounder)						
Swordfish, cooked, dry heat (1 oz)	28	14	4	44	14	33
Trout, Rainbow, cooked, dry heat (1 oz)	28	11	2	43	21	10
Tuna, light, canned in oil, drained solids (1 oz)	28	21	4	56	5	100
Tuna, light, canned in water, drained solids (1 oz)	28	1	1	37	—	101
Tuna, white, canned in oil, drained solids (1 oz)	28	21	—	53	9	112
Tuna, white, canned in water, drained solids (1 oz)	28	6	2	39	12	111
Tuna salad, prepared with light tuna in oil, pickle relish, salad dressing, onion, celery (½ cup)	103	86	14	192	14	412

* *Regular lox has approximately 567 mg sodium per oz.*
** *Value is product with salt added.*

	Weight (g)	Fat (cals)	Sat. Fatty Acids (cals)	Total (cals)	Choles. (mg)	Na (mg)
SHELLFISH						
Clam, cooked, moist heat (1 oz)	28	5	1	42	19	32
Crab, Alaskan King, cooked, moist heat (1 oz)	28	4	tr	27	15	304
Crab, Alaskan King, imitation, made from surimi (1 oz)	28	4	—	29	6	238
Crab, Blue, cooked, moist heat (1 oz)	28	5	1	29	28	79
Crab Cakes, prepared with egg, fried in margarine (1 cake)	60	41	8	93	90	198
Crayfish, cooked, moist heat (1 oz)	28	4	1	32	50	19
Lobster, Northern, cooked, moist heat (1 oz)	28	2	tr	28	20	108
Oyster, Eastern, cooked, breaded and fried (1 oz)	28	32	8	56	23	118
Shrimp, cooked (1 oz)	28	3	1	28	55	63
Shrimp, breaded and fried (4 large)	30	33	5	73	53	103
Shrimp, imitation, made from surimi (1 oz)	28	4	—	29	10	200
Scallop, breaded and fried (2 large)	31	31	7	67	19	144
CHICKEN						
Light meat, without skin, stewed (1 oz)	28	10	3	45	22	18
with skin, stewed (1 oz)	28	25	7	57	21	18
Dark meat, without skin, stewed (1 oz)	28	23	6	54	25	21
with skin, stewed (1 oz)	28	38	14	66	23	20
Breast, half, meat only, stewed (3 oz)	95	26	7	144	73	59
meat and skin, stewed (4 oz)	110	74	21	202	83	68
fried with batter, meat and skin (5 oz)	140	177	44	364	119	385
Drumstick, meat only, stewed (1½ oz)	46	24	6	78	40	37
meat and skin, stewed (2 oz)	57	55	15	116	48	43
fried with batter, meat and skin (2½ oz)	72	101	27	193	62	194
Thigh, meat only, stewed (2 oz)	55	49	14	107	49	41
meat and skin, stewed (2½ oz)	68	90	25	158	57	49
fried with batter, meat and skin (3 oz)	86	128	34	238	80	248

	Weight (g)	Fat (cals)	Sat. Fatty Acids (cals)	Total (cals)	Choles. (mg)	Na (mg)
Chicken *cont.*						
Wing, meat only, stewed (1 oz)	24	15	5	43	18	18
meat and skin, stewed (1½ oz)	40	60	17	100	28	27
fried with batter, meat and						
skin (1¾ oz)	49	96	26	159	39	157
Boneless, canned in broth (1 oz)	28	20	5	47	62	143
Frankfurter, chicken (1 oz)	28	50	14	73	28	388
Giblets—gizzard, heart, liver						
(1 each)						
(2½ oz)	68	32	10	112	243	40
(1 oz)	28	14	5	47	101	17
Liver pâté, canned (2 tbsp)	28	33	—	57	—	—
Roll, chicken, light (1 oz)	28	19	5	45	14	166
Spread, chicken, canned (1 oz)	28	30	—	55	—	—
TURKEY						
Light meat						
meat only, roasted (1 oz)	28	3	1	40	24	16
meat and skin, roasted (1 oz)	28	22	6	46	22	18
Dark meat						
meat only, roasted (1 oz)	28	11	4	46	32	22
meat and skin roasted (1 oz)	28	30	9	63	25	22
Turkey Ham, cured, thigh meat						
(1 oz)	28	13	5	37	—	283
Pastrami (1 oz)	28	16	5	40	—	297
Roll, light and dark meat						
(1 oz)	28	18	5	42	16	166
Frozen with gravy, 1 pkg						
(5 oz)	142	33	11	95	—	786
(1 oz)	28	7	2	19	—	157
Giblets—gizzard, heart, liver						
(1 each)						
(5½ oz)	158	72	22	264	660	92
(1 oz)	28	13	4	47	119	17
GAME						
Goose, domesticated						
meat only, roasted (1 oz)	28	32	12	67	26	20
meat and skin, roasted (1 oz)	28	56	18	86	26	20
BEEF						
Lean only, avg. all grades,						
cooked (1 oz)	28	26	10	63	25	18
Lean only, "Select" grade,						
cooked (1 oz)	28	23	9	60	25	18

	Weight (g)	Fat (cals)	Sat. Fatty Acids (cals)	Total (cals)	Choles. (mg)	Na (mg)
Lean only, "Choice" grade, cooked (1 oz)	28	27	11	64	25	18
Lean only, "Prime" grade, cooked (1 oz)	28	34	14	71	25	18
Flank steak, lean only, broiled (1 oz)	28	38	16	69	20	19
Round steak, lean only, broiled (1 oz)	28	21	7	55	23	18
Top loin steak, lean only, broiled (1 oz)	28	24	10	59	22	19
Rib-eye steak, lean only, broiled (1 oz)	28	30	13	64	23	19
Chuck roast or steak, lean only, braised (1 oz)	28	26	10	66	28	19
Tenderloin, lean only, broiled (1 oz)	28	24	10	59	24	18
Arm roast or steak, lean only, braised (1 oz)	28	26	10	66	28	19
Brain, simmered (1 oz)	28	32	7	45	582	34
Ground beef, extra lean, broiled (1 oz)	28	41	16	75	28	23
lean, broiled (1 oz)	28	45	18	79	29	25
regular, broiled (1 oz)	28	50	20	83	29	26
Heart, simmered (1 oz)	28	14	5	49	55	18
Kidney, simmered (1 oz)	28	9	3	41	110	38
Liver, braised (1 oz)	28	13	5	46	110	30
Shortribs, lean only, braised (1 oz)	28	46	20	84	26	17
Tongue, simmered (1 oz)	28	53	23	80	30	17
Tripe (1 oz)	28	10	5	28	27	13
VEAL						
Arm steak, braised (1 oz)	28	13	3	55	45	27
Blade steak, braised (1 oz)	28	14	4	56	46	30
Loin chop, braised (1 oz)	28	22	6	64	46	25
Rib roast, cooked (1 oz)	28	16	5	48	36	29
LAMB						
Fore shank, braised (1 oz)	28	15	4	53	29	21
Leg, shank portion, roasted (1 oz)	28	17	5	51	25	19
Loin chops, broiled (1 oz)	28	24	9	61	27	24
Rack rib, roasted (1 oz)	28	34	11	66	25	23

	Weight (g)	Fat (cals)	Sat. Fatty Acids (cals)	Total (cals)	Choles. (mg)	Na (mg)
PORK						
Bacon, pan-fried, 4½ slices (1 oz)	28	126	45	163	24	452
Canadian bacon, grilled (1 oz)	28	22	7	52	16	438
Chitterlings, simmered (1 oz)	28	74	26	86	41	11
Fresh pork, lean only						
center loin, fresh, broiled (1 oz)	28	27	9	65	28	22
shoulder, arm picnic, roasted (1 oz)	28	32	11	65	27	23
shoulder, Boston blade, roasted (1 oz)	28	43	14	73	28	21
sirloin, fresh, broiled (1 oz)	28	35	12	69	28	17
tenderloin, roasted (1 oz)	28	13	5	47	26	19
whole leg, roasted (1 oz)	28	28	10	62	27	18
Ham, boneless						
extra lean, roasted (1 oz)	28	14	5	41	15	341
canned, extra lean, roasted (1 oz)	28	13	5	39	8	322
canned, regular, roasted (1 oz)	28	39	13	64	17	267
Liver, braised (1 oz)	28	12	4	47	101	14
Spareribs, lean and fat, braised (1 oz)	28	77	30	113	34	26
LUNCHEON MEAT AND SAUSAGE						
Bologna, beef and pork (1 oz)	28	72	27	89	16	289
Braunschweiger, pork (1 oz)	28	82	28	102	44	324
Chicken spread, canned (2 tbsp)	26	30	—	55	—	—
Frankfurter						
beef and pork (1 oz)	28	75	28	91	14	318
chicken (1 oz)	28	50	14	73	28	388
Pepperoni, pork, beef (1 oz)	28	113	41	141	—	578
Salad spread, ham, cured (2 tbsp)	30	42	14	64	12	274
Salami, dry, pork, beef (1 oz)	28	88	32	119	22	527
Sausage						
Italian, pork, cooked (1 oz)	28	66	23	92	22	261
knockwurst, pork, beef (1 oz)	28	71	26	87	16	286
pork, fresh, cooked (1 oz)	28	79	28	105	24	366
liverwurst, pork (1 oz)	28	73	27	93	45	244
Polish, pork (1 oz)	28	73	26	92	20	248
Vienna, beef and pork, canned (1½ link)	28	64	24	79	15	270

	Weight (g)	Fat (cals)	Sat. Fatty Acids (cals)	Total (cals)	Choles. (mg)	Na (mg)
MIXED DISHES WITH MEAT, POULTRY, AND SEAFOOD						
Chicken à la king (1 cup)	245	309	116	468	220	760
Chicken and noodle casserole (1 cup)	240	167	53	367	—	600
Chili con carne, w/beans, canned (1 cup)	255	140	68	339	—	1354
Chop suey, beef and pork, without noodles (1 cup)	250	153	77	300	—	1053
Chow mein, chicken, without noodles (1 cup)	250	90	22	255	—	718
Macaroni and cheese, homemade (1 cup)	200	200	107	430	—	1086
canned (1 cup)	240	86	38	228	—	730
Pâté, chicken liver (2 tbsp)	26	31	—	52	—	—
Pizza, cheese (1 slice)	120	77	38	290	56	698
pepperoni (1 slice)	120	104	—	306	—	817
Pot pie, chicken (⅓ of 9″ diameter)	232	282	93	545	56	594
beef (⅓ of 9″ diameter)	210	275	71	517	42	596
Spaghetti with meatballs and tomato sauce, canned (1 cup)	250	97	20	258	—	1220
Stew, beef and vegetable (1 cup)	245	95	40	218	72	292
FAST FOOD						
Bacon cheeseburger (1)	150	246	—	464	68	660
Burrito (1)	174	122	—	392	56	1030
Cheeseburger: regular (1)	112	136	—	299	45	672
4-oz patty (1)	194	283	—	524	105	1224
Eggs, scrambled (2)	95	132	—	175	346	226
Enchilada (1)	230	188	—	396	—	1332
English-muffin sandwich with egg, cheese, bacon (1)	138	163	—	359	214	832
Fish sandwich, regular with cheese (1)	140	204	—	421	56	668
large (1)	170	240	—	469	90	621
French-fried potatoes (3 oz)	85	128	—	274	14	152
Ham and cheese sandwich (1)	155	144	—	372	70	1118
Hamburger: regular (1)	98	100	36	245	32	463
double meat and double-decker roll (1)	190	266	90	524	78	893
4-oz patty, regular roll	174	190	63	444	71	762
4 oz patty, large roll (1)	264	335	117	668	114	1019

	Weight (g)	Fat (cals)	Sat. Fatty Acids (cals)	Total (cals)	Choles. (mg)	Na (mg)
Fast food cont.						
Hog dog (1)	82	123	45	214	37	636
Hot-fudge sundae (1)	165	98	—	312	18	177
Hushpuppy (3 pieces)	45	50	—	153	—	—
Onion rings (3 oz)	85	140	—	285	16	485
Pancake, butter, syrup (3)	200	94	—	468	46	1020
Roast beef on bun (5 oz)	150	121	36	347	56	756
Taco (1)	81	135	36	187	21	456
Tuna sub (1)	255	250	—	566	—	1288
Turnover, apple (1)	85	127	—	255	4	326
EGGS						
Whole, raw (1)	50	50	15	79	274	69
Yolk, raw (1)	17	50	15	63	272	8
White, raw (1)	33	tr	0	16	0	50
Fried in butter (1)	46	58	22	83	246	144
scrambled with butter and milk (1)	64	64		95	248	155
Egg substitute,* liquid (¼ cup)	60	18	4	50	1	106
frozen (¼ cup)	60	60	11	96	1	120
Omelet with butter and milk (1 egg)	64	64	25	95	248	155
DAIRY PRODUCTS						
MILK						
Buttermilk, cultured (1 cup)	245	20	12	99	9	257
Hot cocoa, with whole milk (1 cup)	250	82	50	218	33	123
Condensed, sweetened, canned (1 cup)	306	239	151	982	104	389
Evaporated, skim, canned (½ cup)	128	3	2	99	5	147
Evaporated, whole, canned (½ cup)	126	86	52	169	37	133
Milk						
skim or nonfat (1 cup)	245	4	3	86	4	126
1% fat (1 cup)	244	23	14	102	10	123
2% fat (1 cup)	244	42	26	121	18	122
whole (1 cup)	244	74	46	150	33	120
whole, chocolate (1 cup)	250	77	48	208	30	149
Milk shake, vanilla, thick (11 oz)	313	86	53	350	37	299

* Check label—several brands are fat-free.

	Weight (g)	Fat (cals)	Sat. Fatty Acids (cals)	Total (cals)	Choles. (mg)	Na (mg)
Malted-milk beverage (1 cup whole milk + 2 to 3 heaping tsp malted-milk powder)	265	89	54	236	37	215
YOGURT						
Nonfat or skim, plain (1 cup)	227	4	3	127	4	174
Low-fat, plain (1 cup)	227	32	21	144	14	159
Whole, plain (1 cup)	227	67	43	139	29	105
FROZEN DESSERTS						
Frozen yogurt (½ cup)	113	21	14	123	9	60
Ice cream, rich, 16% fat (½ cup)	74	106	67	175	44	54
Ice cream, regular, 10% fat (½ cup)	67	67	41	135	30	58
Ice milk, regular (½ cup)	66	25	16	92	9	53
Ice milk, soft serve (½ cup)	88	21	13	112	7	82
Sherbet, orange (½ cup)	97	17	11	135	7	44
CREAM, NONDAIRY CREAMERS, AND TOPPINGS						
Creamer, nondairy, liquid (1 tbsp)	15	14	3	20	0	12
Creamer, nondairy, powder (1 tsp)	2	6	6	11	0	4
Half-&-half cream (1 tbsp)	15	15	10	20	6	6
Sour cream, real (1 tbsp)	12	23	14	26	5	6
Whipped cream, pressurized (1 tbsp)	3	6	4	8	2	4
Dessert topping, nondairy, frozen (1 tbsp)	4	9	8	13	0	1
Whipping cream, heavy, fluid (1 tbsp)	15	50	32	52	21	6
CHEESE*						
American (1 oz)	28	80	50	106	27	406
Blue, Brie, Cheddar, Colby, Edam, Gouda, Gruyère, Monterey, Parmesan, Roquefort, Swiss (1 oz)	28	85	54	114	30	176
Cheese spread, process, American (1 oz)	28	54	34	82	16	381
Cottage cheese, dry curd (½ cup)	73	3	2	62	5	10
low-fat, 1% fat (½ cup)	113	11	6	82	5	459
low-fat, 2% fat (½ cup)	113	20	13	101	9	459
creamed (½ cup)	105	42	27	109	16	425

* *Many low-fat varieties are in grocery stores—check label.*

	Weight (g)	Fat (cals)	Sat. Fatty Acids (cals)	Total (cals)	Choles. (mg)	Na (mg)
Cheese *cont.*						
Cream cheese, regular (1 oz)	28	89	56	99	31	84
Cream cheese, Neufachâtel (1 oz)	28	59	38	74	22	113
Mozzarella, part skim (1 oz)	28	41	26	72	16	132
Ricotta, part skim milk (1 oz)	28	20	13	39	9	35
Ricotta, whole milk (1 oz)	28	33	22	49	14	24
FATS						
OIL						
Canola (1 tsp)	5	40	3	40	0	0
Corn (1 tsp)	5	40	5	40	0	0
Olive (1 tsp)	5	40	5	40	0	0
Peanut (1 tsp)	5	40	7	40	0	0
Safflower (1 tsp)	5	40	4	40	0	0
Sesame (1 tsp)	5	40	5	40	0	0
Soybean (1 tsp)	5	40	6	40	0	0
Soybean/cottonseed (1 tsp)	5	40	7	40	0	0
Soybean, hydrogenated (1 tsp)	5	40	6	40	0	0
Sunflower (1 tsp)	5	40	4	40	0	0
MARGARINE						
Corn oil stick (1 tsp)	5	34	5	34	0	44
Corn oil, tub (1 tsp)	5	34	6	34	0	51
Diet (2 tsp)	10	33	5	33	0	92
Safflower oil, tub (1 tsp)	5	34	4	34	0	51
Soybean, hydrogenated, tub (1 tsp)	5	34	5	34	0	51
Soybean, hydrogenated, whipped, tub (1 tsp)	5	26	5	26	0	48
NUTS (approx. 3 tbsp)						
Almonds, dried	28	133	13	167	0	3
Brazil nuts, dried	28	169	41	186	0	0
Cashews, dry roasted	28	119	23	163	0	4
Chestnuts, roasted	28	3	1	68	0	1
Coconut, flaked, sweetened	28	81	72	126	0	76
Filberts/hazelnuts, dried	28	160	12	179	0	1
Macadamia nuts, oil roasted	28	195	30	204	0	2
Mixed nuts, dry roasted	28	131	18	169	0	3
Peanuts, oil roasted	28	126	17	165	0	4
Pecans, dried	28	173	14	190	0	0
Pistachios, dry roasted	28	135	17	172	0	2
Walnuts, English, dried	28	158	14	182	0	3
Walnuts, Black	28	145	9	172	0	0

	Weight (g)	Fat (cals)	Sat. Fatty Acids (cals)	Total (cals)	Choles. (mg)	Na (mg)
SEEDS (approx. 3 tbsp)						
Pumpkin, squash, dried	28	117	23	154	0	5
Sesame, roasted & toasted	28	122	17	161	0	3
Sunflower, dried	28	127	14	162	0	1
SALAD DRESSING						
Blue cheese (1 tbsp)	15	72	14	77	—	—
French (1 tbsp)	16	58	14	67	—	214
Italian (1 tbsp)	15	64	9	69	0	116
Mayonnaise (1 tbsp)	14	99	14	99	8	78
Mayonnaise type (1 tbsp)	15	44	6	57	4	104
Thousand Island (1 tbsp)	16	50	8	59	5	109
Vinegar and oil (1 tbsp)	16	72	14	72	0	0
Sandwich spread, commercial (1 tbsp)	15	47	7	60	12	—
OTHER FATS						
Butter (1 tsp)	5	36	23	36	11	41
Olives, green (10 small)	34	32	4	33	0	686
Olives, ripe (5 extra large)	28	30	4	30	0	193
Peanut butter, smooth (2 tsp)	11	50	8	63	0	52
Shortening, hydrogenated soybean and cottenseed (1 tsp)	4	38	10	38	0	—
BREAD, CEREALS, PASTA, AND STARCHY VEGETABLES						
BREADS, PANCAKES, AND WAFFLES						
Bagel, 3″ diameter (1)	100	23	—	296	—	360
Biscuit, made with milk, 2″ diameter (1)	28	23	5.4	91	—	272
Bread, white (1 slice)	23	8	2	63	—	114
Bun, hamburger, 3½″ diameter, or hot dog, 6″ long (1)	40	20	5	119	—	202
English muffin, plain (half)	29	5	—	69	—	185
French toast (1 slice)	65	60	—	153	—	257
Muffin, bran, 2″ diameter bottom (1)	40	35	11	104	—	179
Pancake, with egg, milk, 6″ diameter × ½″ thick (1)	73	48	17	164	—	412
Popover, 2¾″ top, 2″ bottom, 4″ high in center (1)	40	33	12	90	—	88
Roll, hard, 3¾″ diameter × 2″ high (1)	50	14	4	156	—	313
Waffle, 9″ × 9″ × ⅝″ square (1)	200	176	57	558	—	290

	Weight (g)	Fat (cals)	Sat. Fatty Acids (cals)	Total (cals)	Choles. (mg)	Na (mg)
CEREALS, READY-TO-EAT						
40% bran flakes (1 oz)	28	5	0	93	0	264
Corn flakes (1 oz)	28	1	0	110	0	351
Granola, homemade (1 oz)	28	69	13	138	—	3
Grapenuts (1 oz)	28	1	0	101	0	197
Puffed wheat, plain (1 oz)	28	4	0	104	0	2
Shredded wheat (1 large biscuit)	24	3	0	83	0	0
Wheat germ, plain, toasted						
(1 oz)	28	27	5	108	0	1
CEREALS, COOKED						
Corn grits, regular and quick						
(1 cup)	242	5	0	146	0	0 *
Cream of wheat, regular (1 cup)	251	5	0	134	0	2 *
Oatmeal, regular, quick and						
instant (1 cup)	234	22	4	145	0	1 *
PASTA AND RICE, COOKED						
Noodles, chow mein, canned						
(1 cup)	45	95	18	220	5	450
Noodles, egg (1 cup)	160	22	—	200	50	3 *
Rice, white, brown, or wild						
(1 cup)	205	2	0	223	0	4 *
Spaghetti (1 cup)	140	5	0	155	—	1 *
STARCHY VEGETABLES						
Corn, lima beans, green peas,						
plantain, white potato,						
winter or acorn squash, yam						
or sweet potato (½ cup)	—	0	0	80	0	**
PREPARED VEGETABLES						
Coleslaw/dressing with table						
cream (½ cup)	60	14	2	42	5	14
Corn pudding, whole milk, egg,						
butter (½ cup)	125	59	28	136	115	69
French fries						
oven-heated, cottage-cut (10)	50	37	17	109	0	23
fried in animal and						
veg. fat (10)	50	75	31	158	6	108
Onion rings, frozen,						
oven-heated (7)	70	168	54	285	0	263
Potato chips (1 oz)	28	91	23	148	0	133

* *Product cooked in unsalted water.*
** *Canned vegetables are high in sodium unless label states canned without salt.*

	Weight (g)	Fat (cals)	Sat. Fatty Acids (cals)	Total (cals)	Choles. (mg)	Na (mg)
Potato						
au gratin with whole milk, butter, and cheese (½ cup)	122	84	52	160	29	528
hashed brown, in oil (½ cup)	78	98	38	163	—	19
mashed, whole milk, margarine (½ cup)	105	40	10	111	2	309
O'Brien, whole milk, butter (½ cup)	97	12	7	79	4	211
scalloped, whole milk, butter (½ cup)	122	41	25	105	14	409
salad, egg, mayonnaise (½ cup)	125	93	16	179	86	661
pancake, eggs, margarine (1)	76	113	31	495	93	388
potato sticks (1 oz)	28	88	23	148	0	71
potato puff, vegetable oil (½ cup)	62	60	29	138	0	462
candied sweet potatoes, brown sugar, butter, 2½″ × 2″ piece (1)	105	31	13	144	8	73
SOUP, CANNED						
Bean with bacon, prepared with water (1 cup)	253	53	14	173	3	952
Beef broth or bouillon, ready-to-serve (1 cup)	240	5	3	16	tr	782
Beef, chunky style, ready-to-serve (1 cup)	240	46	23	171	14	867
Chicken broth, prepared with water (1 cup)	244	13	4	39	1	776
Chicken, chunky style, ready-to-serve (1 cup)	251	59	18	178	30	887
Chicken noodle, prepared with water (1 cup)	241	23	6	75	7	1107
Chicken rice, prepared with water (1 cup)	241	17	5	60	7	814
Chili beef, prepared with water (1 cup)	250	59	30	169	12	1035
Cream of chicken, prepared with water (1 cup)	244	67	19	116	10	986
Cream of mushroom, prepared with water (1 cup)	244	81	22	129	2	1031
Gazpacho, ready-to-serve (1 cup)	244	20	3	57	0	1183
Minestrone, prepared with water (1 cup)	241	23	5	83	2	911

	Weight (g)	Fat (cals)	Sat. Fatty Acids (cals)	Total (cals)	Choles. (mg)	Na (mg)
Soup, canned *cont.*						
Oyster stew, prepared with water (1 cup)	241	34	23	59	14	980
Split pea with ham, prepared with water (1 cup)	253	40	16	189	8	1008
Tomato, prepared with water (1 cup)	244	17	4	86	0	872
Tomato rice, prepared with water (1 cup)	247	24	5	120	2	815
Vegetarian vegetable, prepared with water (1 cup)	241	17	3	72	0	823
CRACKERS						
Bread sticks, 7½″ × ¾″ diameter (5)	25	7	2	96	0	175
Cheese crackers (10)	31	60	23	150	—	325
Graham crackers, 2½″ sq. (4 squares)	28	23	5	110	—	190
Saltines (10 crackers)	28	31	7	123	—	312
Zwieback crackers (4 pieces)	28	25	10	121	6	66
Sandwich-type, cheese-peanut butter (4 sandwiches)	28	61	16	139	—	281
BAKING INGREDIENTS						
Cornmeal, dry (1 cup)	138	15	—	502	—	1
Cornstarch, not packed (1 tbsp)	8	tr	0	29	—	tr
Flour, white (1 cup)	115	11	—	419	—	2
VEGETABLES AND FRUITS						
VEGETABLES						
All vegetables are low in fat and saturated fat (½–1 cup)	—	2	0	25	0	*
FRUIT						
Apple, raw, 2¾″ diameter (1)	138	5	1	81	0	1
Applesauce, canned, unsweetened (½ cup)	122	1	0	53	0	2
Apricots, medium, raw (4)	141	5	0	68	0	1
Banana, 9″ long (half)	57	3	1	53	0	1
Blackberries, raw (¾ cup)	108	4	0	56	0	0
Cantaloupe (1 cup, cubes)	160	4	0	57	0	14
Cherries, sweet, raw (12)	82	7	2	59	0	0
Figs, medium, raw (2)	100	3	0	74	0	2
Fruit cocktail, canned, juice packed (½ cup)	124	1	0	56	0	4

* *Sodium values vary from 2 to 63 mg per ½ cup cooked.*
  Canned vegetables are higher in sodium than fresh or frozen.

	Weight (g)	Fat (cals)	Sat. Fatty Acids (cals)	Total (cals)	Choles. (mg)	Na (mg)
Grapefruit (half)	123	1	0	37	0	0
Grapes, raw (15)	36	1	0	23	0	0
Honeydew melon (1 cup, cubes)	170	2	0	60	0	17
Kiwifruit (1 large)	91	4	0	55	0	4
Mango, raw (half)	104	3	0	68	0	2
Nectarine, 2½" diameter (1)	136	5	0	67	0	0
Orange, 2½" diameter (1)	131	2	0	62	0	0
Papaya (1 cup, cubes)	140	2	1	54	0	4
Peach, 2½" diameter (1)	87	1	0	37	0	0
Peaches, canned, water packed (2 halves)	154	1	0	36	0	6
Pear, raw (1)	166	6	0	98	0	1
Pineapple, raw (¾ cup)	116	5	0	58	0	2
Pineapple, canned, juice pack (⅓ cup)	83	1	0	50	0	1
Plum, raw, 2⅛" diameter (2)	132	6	1	72	0	0
Pomegranate (half)	77	2	0	52	0	3
Raspberries, raw (1 cup)	123	6	0	61	0	0
Strawberries, raw, whole (1¼ cup)	186	6	0	56	0	3
Tangerine, 2½" diameter (2)	168	3	0	74	0	2
Watermelon (1¼ cup, cubes)	200	8	0	63	0	4
DRIED FRUIT						
Apples, uncooked (4 rings)	26	1	0	62	0	22
Apricots, uncooked (7 halves)	25	1	0	58	0	2
Dates (2½)	21	1	0	57	0	1
Figs, uncooked (1½)	28	3	1	72	0	3
Prunes, uncooked (3)	25	1	0	60	0	1
Raisins (2 tbsp)	21	1	0	62	0	2
FRUIT JUICE						
Apple juice (½ cup)	124	1	0	58	0	4
Cranberry juice cocktail (⅓ cup)	84	0	0	49	0	3
Grapefruit juice, unsweetened (½ cup)	124	1	0	47	0	2
Grape juice (⅓ cup)	84	1	0	52	0	2
Orange juice (½ cup)	125	3	0	55	0	1
Pineapple juice (½ cup)	125	1	0	70	0	1
Prune juice (⅓ cup)	85	0	0	60	0	4

DESSERTS AND SNACKS
CAKES, COOKIES, PIES, AND OTHER BAKED GOODS

	Weight (g)	Fat (cals)	Sat. Fatty Acids (cals)	Total (cals)	Choles. (mg)	Na (mg)
Brownies, with nuts and icing (⅙ of 7½" × 5¼" × ⅞" pan)	60	113	39	257	—	123

	Weight (g)	Fat (cals)	Sat. Fatty Acids (cals)	Total (cals)	Choles. (mg)	Na (mg)
Cakes, cookies, pies, and other baked goods *cont.*						
Cake, without frosting						
angel food (⅟₁₂ of						
10″ diameter)	60	1	0	161	0	170
devil's food, sheet cake						
(3″ × 3″ × 2″ piece)	88	136	—	322	41	259
white, 2-layer (⅟₁₆ of						
9″ diameter)	53	77	20	198	3	171
Boston cream pie, 2-layer						
(⅟₁₂ of 8″ diameter)	69	59	18	208	—	128
fruitcake (⅟₃₂ of						
7″ diameter)	43	64	14	167	60	83
pound cake (⅟₁₂ of						
8½″ loaf)	42	70	18	171	32	74
sponge cake (⅟₁₂ of						
9¾″ diameter)	66	34	11	196	7	110
yellow, 2-layer (⅟₁₆ of						
9″ diameter)	54	62	17	197	36	140
Cake frosting						
chocolate, prepared with						
milk and fat (1 tbsp.)	17	22	12	65	—	11
coconut with boiled						
frosting (1 tbsp.)	10	7	6	38	—	12
fudge made with water						
(from mix) (1 tbsp.)	15	9	3	52	—	36
white boiled (1 tbsp.)	6	0	0	19	0	8
Cheesecake (1 portion)	100	173	—	302	170	222
Cookies, sandwich,						
1¾″ diameter (4)	40	81	22	198	—	193
chocolate chip,						
2⅓″ diameter (4)	40	108	31	206	—	139
fig bars (4)	56	28	8	200	—	141
gingersnaps,						
2″ diameter (4)	28	23	5	118	—	160
Cupcake, plain, no icing,						
2½″ diameter (1)	25	32	9	91	—	75
plain, with white uncooked						
icing, 2½″ diameter (1)	35	37	10	128	—	79
Doughnut, cake type,						
3⅝″ diameter (1)	58	97	24	227	—	291
yeast type,						
3¾″ diameter (1)	42	102	25	176	—	99

	Weight (g)	Fat (cals)	Sat. Fatty Acids (cals)	Total (cals)	Choles. (mg)	Na (mg)
Pastry, Danish, plain 4¼″ diameter × 1″ thick (1)	65	138	41	274	—	238
Pastry, toaster, commercial (1)	52	54	—	203	—	239
Pie, apple, 2 crust (⅛ of 9″ diameter)	118	118	31	302	—	355
custard (⅛ of 9″ diameter)	114	114	39	249	—	327
pumpkin (⅛ of 9″ diameter)	114	115	41	241	—	244
pecan (⅛ of 9″ diameter)	103	212	30	431	—	228
cherry, 2 crust (⅛ of 9″ diameter)	118	120	32	308	—	359
Pie crust, baked (⅛ of pie 9″ diameter)	23	68	16	113	—	138
CANDY						
Candy corn (approx. 20 pieces)	28	5	1	103	—	60
Milk chocolate, plain (1 oz)	28	83	46	147	—	27
Milk chocolate, almond (1 oz)	28	91	41	151	—	23
Caramels, plain or chocolate (1 oz)	28	26	14	113	—	64
Chocolate coated peanuts (8–16)	28	105	27	159	—	17
Fudge, plain (1 oz)	28	32	11	113	—	54
Gumdrops (1 oz)	28	2	0	98	0	10
Hard candy (1 oz)	28	3	0	109	0	9
Marshmallow (1 oz)	28	tr	0	90	0	11
Mints (uncoated) (1 oz)	28	5	1	103	0	60
SAUCES AND GRAVIES						
DEHYDRATED SAUCES						
Béarnaise, prepared with milk and butter (¼ cup)	64	154	94	175	47	316
Cheese, prepared with milk (¼ cup)	70	39	21	77	13	92
Hollandaise, prepared with milk and butter (¼ cup)	64	154	95	176	47	284
Mushroom, prepared with milk (¼ cup)	67	23	13	57	9	383
Sour cream, prepared with milk (¼ cup)	79	68	36	127	23	252
Stroganoff, prepared with milk and water (¼ cup)	74	24	15	68	10	457

	Weight (g)	Fat (cals)	Sat. Fatty Acids (cals)	Total (cals)	Choles. (mg)	Na (mg)
Dehydrated sauces *cont.*						
Sweet and sour, prepared with water and vinegar (¼ cup)	78	0	0	74	0	195
White, prepared with milk (¼ cup)	66	31	14	60	9	199
READY-TO-SERVE SAUCES						
Barbecue (¼ cup)	63	10	0	47	0	510
Soy (1 tbsp)	18	0	0	11	0	1029
Teriyaki (1 tbsp)	18	0	0	15	0	690
CANNED GRAVY						
Au jus (¼ cup)	60	1	1	10	0	—
Beef (¼ cup)	58	13	6	31	2	29
Chicken (¼ cup)	60	31	7	47	1	344
Mushroom (¼ cup)	60	14	2	30	0	340
Turkey (½ cup)	60	12	4	31	1	—
DEHYDRATED GRAVY						
Au jus, prepared with water (¼ cup)	62	2	1	5	0	145
Brown, prepared with water (¼ cup)	65	1	0	22	tr	31
Chicken, prepared with water (¼ cup)	65	5	1	21	1	283
Mushroom, prepared with water (¼ cup)	64	2	1	18	0	351
Onion, prepared with water (¼ cup)	65	2	1	20	0	259
Pork, prepared with water (¼ cup)	64	5	2	19	1	309
Turkey, prepared with water (¼ cup)	65	5	1	22	1	375

GETTING THE LEAD OUT

Ways of Reducing Dietary Fat and Cholesterol

4

Since atherosclerosis is largely a disease of life-style, it is necessary to know what and how much a person eats, and what he or she does away from the dinner table. The reversal diet profile is usually revealing—to both me and the patient. Sometimes it is even shocking.

Take the case of the patient I'll call Jim. In keeping a diary he found that his breakfasts usually consisted of whole-wheat toast, margarine and jam, coffee without cream and sugar . . . and two scrambled eggs fried in generous amounts of butter. Lunch was most often a diet soda, salad with low-calorie dressing . . . and deep-fried chicken. Dinner was usually skim milk, vegetables of one sort or another . . . and steak with gravy, or roast meat, or pan-fried chicken. Snacks and desserts were always chocolate bars or ice cream. Most days he had a couple of cocktails, too.

The facts shown by the diet diary shocked Jim. There were days in which he was taking in 900 milligrams of cholesterol, at least three times the amount of cholesterol now recommended by the American Heart Association.

The diary was an eye-opener for Jim. "No wonder my cholesterol count is 280," he said to me in my office one day.

This moment of revelation for Jim was immediately followed by another. "So what am I supposed to eat?" Good question.

Life in our deep-fried society is sometimes like being adrift in a sea of saturated fats and cholesterol. Unless you know what to look for, the question, "What am I suppose to eat?" can often be followed with the one-word answer, "Nothing."

But there are comfortable ways around abstinence. There are "good" and satisfying foods that can lower cholesterol and help reverse heart disease risks. There are even changes that can be made that won't change the flavor of food but will alter the effect it has in your body. There are wonderful foods that can make you lose weight, lower total cholesterol, raise the blood's HDL levels, and gobble up LDLs.

And as you now know when blood cholesterol is lowered, heart disease can be halted or reversed.

I have seen the immediate effects of reducing saturated fats and dietary cholesterol in my own studies. To examine fat content in blood I fed one group of people a meal that was low in fat and high in carbohydrates. Another group of test subjects was fed a meal of equal calories that was high in saturated fats: a hamburger, milk shake, and french fries.

After a couple of hours to give the food time to digest, I drew a test tube of blood from the subjects in each test group and spun it down in a centrifuge to force the red and white blood cells and the platelets to the tube's bottom.

The clear fluid left on top—the *plasma*—of the carbohydrate eaters was relatively clear. But the plasma of the fat eaters was clouded with globules of fat. The difference in clarity was almost like placing a glass of beer next to a milk shake.

To remove cholesterol and saturated fats from your diet, you first have to find them.

Cholesterol and Fat

As far as your cardiovascular system is concerned, the building blocks of atherosclerosis come in two forms: fat and cholesterol. Generally speaking, when you look for something to blame in heart disease, the finger can be pointed at those two elements.

The surgeon general did just that in his *Report on Nutrition and Health* when he concluded that "overconsumption of certain dietary components [saturated fat and cholesterol] is now a major concern for Americans."

His report and other government studies have pointed out that about 37 percent of our calories come from fat, well over the 30 percent recommended by the American Heart Association. More than half of that fat comes from saturated sources such as meat and dairy products, and more subtle sources such as the coconut oils and palm-kernel oils found in processed foods. What effect does high consumption of saturated fats have on the rate of heart disease? Dr. Ancel Keys and associates analyzed dietary habits in seven countries and found a direct link between the intake of saturated fat and the incidence of heart disease.

At least we eat better today than we did in the late 1950s, when about 70 percent of the fat in our daily diet came from animal sources. Heart disease is still the top killer in this country, but now we are struggling to reverse its deadly effects. We are among the countries most afflicted by this disease, but we are leading the world in reversing its course.

Still, as any cardiologist will tell you, we have a long way to go in our fight against heart disease. And much of the blame goes to the things we eat. After years of examining the diet diaries of coronary heart disease patients, I have come to several conclusions about people and their eating habits.

• *Most people are astounded by how much they eat:* Honest food diaries generally produce honest amazement: "I didn't realize I ate that much!" When every handful of peanuts is written down, when every potato chip and every piece of chocolate candy are committed to paper, this "background" eating can often equal an extra meal filled with fat calories and extra cholesterol. After keeping a diet diary, most people realize how easy it is to overeat in our society, where food is plentiful.

• *Most people will make long-term changes if they are given replacements for "bad" foods:* Most everyone can make short-term changes. That is what the phenomenon known as "yo-yo dieting" is all about, in which people radically change eating habits long enough to lose ten or twenty pounds and then sinfully revert to their old ways of eating and gain it all back.

The best way to make effective changes is to find satisfying substitutes for high-fat, high-cholesterol foods and to make changes slowly. That way you don't have to reverse your life-style in order to reverse the numbers that lead to heart disease.

• *The changes necessary to reduce saturated fats and dietary cholesterol are usually surprisingly small:* The culprits in the diets of many of my patients have been just one or two items. Or maybe the foods they eat aren't bad in themselves, but the way they are prepared is raising their saturated fat intake.

For instance, after analyzing your diet diary, you may see that your cholesterol intake is well within the 300 milligrams or less cholesterol that is allowed under the reversal diet, *except* for the two eggs per day you are eating. Those two eggs will add almost 600 milligrams of extra cholesterol.

How to get rid of them without dietary inconvenience? Try yolkless egg recipes, or ones that incorporate egg substitutes. That way you can have your eggs and lower cholesterol, too.

The Saturated Villain

Although total dietary fat has been singled out as a villain of our arteries, the real culprit is saturated fat.

Foods with dietary cholesterol always have saturated fats in them. But foods containing saturated fats don't always contain cholesterol. For example, tropical oils like coconut oil, palm oil, and cocoa butter which are used in commercial products, are rich in saturated fats even though they are free of cholesterol.

This is particularly bad because it allows processed-food companies to advertise their products as being "cholesterol free," giving the impression that these foods are harmless.

Many shortenings, cookies, crackers, coffee creamers, and even oat-bran cereals which have become so popular because they lower cholesterol contain hearty doses of these saturated fats from tropical oils. These foods contain no cholesterol. But if they contain a substance such as palm-kernel oil, which has been shown to raise cholesterol levels, then it is nothing short of dishonest (not to mention dangerous) to imply that these foods are free of heart-harming agents. That's because foods high in saturated fat cause elevated cholesterol levels in the blood when the fats are processed in the body.

Some common sources of saturated fats without cholesterol are:

> **Cocoa butter**
> **Coconut**
> **Coconut oil**
> **Hydrogenated vegetable oil**
> **Partially hydrogenated vegetable oil**
> **Palm-kernel oil**
> **Shortening**
> **Vegetable oil (if it contains palm or coconut oil)**

Although the naked eye may have trouble spotting saturated fats, your liver has no problem at all. It produces cholesterol-rich bile which serves to digest fats. But because saturated fats are such complex molecules, more bile has to be produced to do the job of digestion than with unsaturated fats.

Much of the extra cholesterol in this bile circulates in the bloodstream where it bonds with saturated fat.

Also, for reasons not understood, saturated fat reduces the number of LDL receptors in the liver. These receptors serve to pull LDL cholesterol from the bloodstream, but if they aren't there to perform that function, this dangerous LDL continues to build up.

Unsaturated fats, on the other hand, require less bile for digestion. They also bind with the cholesterol and pass into the intestines instead of the bloodstream. Research conducted by Dr. Grace Goldsmith and published in the *Archives of Internal Medicine* shows that an unsaturated-fat diet leads to 20 to 25 percent more bile being eliminated from the body than does a saturated-fat diet. This, in turn, means lower levels of cholesterol in the bloodstream.

In short: *Saturated fats raise total cholesterol,* while *unsaturated fats lower total cholesterol.*

The message here is clear. To help reverse or stop coronary heart disease, favor unsaturated fats in your diet.

THE SATURATED-FAT GOAL:
10 Percent of Calories or Less

The 1987 report of the panel that formed the National Cholesterol Education Program is the culmination of millions of dollars, thousands of man-hours, and decades of dedicated research spent in determining the optimal diet for the American public. Much (if not most) of this research has been aimed at answering questions about fat levels in the diet: How much total fat should you eat? What kind of fat should it be?

This blue-ribbon panel of medical researchers says that 30 percent or less of your daily diet should consist of fat. But 10 percent *or less* of your total calories should consist of saturated fats. A reduction to less than 7 percent is recommended if total cholesterol (and LDL cholesterol) doesn't reach the proper level after three months.

On the surface, this represents a major shift in eating patterns for a country in which about 18 percent of our total calories come from saturated fats. But actually, as you will see in the pages ahead, dramatic reductions in the amount of saturated fat you eat might not require dramatic changes. The advice in the rest of this chapter is the culmination of years of suggestions given patients who ask the question: "How can I get fat and cholesterol out of my diet?"

Here are some guidelines:

• *Reduce fat in recipes by one-half:* If a recipe calls for the addition of four tablespoons of oil, add two instead, making up for the rest of the oil by adding two more tablespoons of water. Don't forget to use polyunsaturated oils such as corn or safflower.

• *Bake without yolks:* To get the cholesterol of the egg yolk out of baked goods, just use the egg whites. Substitute a teaspoonful of polyunsaturated oil for each yolk that you don't use.

• *Down with deep-fried breads:* If you must eat doughnuts, make them the baked variety. Deep-fried breads act like a sponge to the oil they are cooked in, soaking it up and eventually depositing it in your arteries. Many doughnut shops fry their breads in cooking oil that contains saturated fat, which makes them much worse than even their corn-oil-fried cousins.

• *Beware of lard, coconut, palm oil, or shortening:* While we're on the subject of bakery goods, watch out for the above-mentioned oils in commercially baked goods. Baked goods prepared with vegetable oils other than those mentioned above are best.

• *Trade coffee creamers for skim or dried low-fat milk:* Creamers usually contain coconut oils, which are high in saturated fats. Most coffee creamers contain a large percentage of saturated fat. Skim milk, on the other hand, contains almost no saturated fat.

• *Substitute skim milk for whole milk, whole milk for cream:* One cup of skim milk contains a scant 4 milligrams of cholesterol and 0.0 grams of fat, whereas one cup of whole milk contains 30 milligrams of cholesterol and 9 grams of fat. One-half cup half-and-half contains a whopping 96 milligrams of cholesterol and 28 grams of fat. These substitutions can represent big differences in your diet with little sacrifice.

There is no question that drinking milk is very important to maintain a healthy heart and to prevent osteoporosis. An examination of the dietary habits of 60,000 women in the Nurses Health Study showed that a daily calcium intake of 800 milligrams and above offers a 23 percent reduction in the risk of developing hypertension. Another study of equal magnitude by the National Center for Health Statistics suggested that a daily calcium intake of 400 to 600 milligrams greatly lowers the risk of high blood pressure.

Since a normal blood pressure is one of the most important reversal goals, I think it is important to drink your milk in order to get this daily dose of calcium. Just drink your milk nonfat.

• *Use really light cheeses:* You can also get a healthy portion of calcium from cheese. Just make sure it's *really* light.

Cheese labeled as being "light" may actually contain less fat than the regular variety, but it can still be "heavy" with fat. An ounce of some types of cheese that contain 50 percent fat may still contain a whopping 5 grams of fat, meaning that about 60 percent of its calories come from fat.

But there are some low-fat cheeses on the market that are truly low in fat. Here are three of the best:

• *Hoop cheese:* Sometimes called "baker's cheese" because it is often used by bakers, this soft cheese contains less than a gram of fat and 10 milligrams of sodium per ounce. It is good in cooked dishes as well as in dips and spreads.

Hoop cheese has an acidic taste because of the way it is produced, with the curd being separated from the whey without being cooked or washed. If you can't find this cheese in your market, it can be approximated by rinsing low-fat cottage cheese in cold water.

• *Gammelost:* This semisoft cheese from Norway contains about 0.3 grams of fat and 85 milligrams of sodium per ounce. It has a bluish cast to it and a sharp flavor. It is low in fat because it is made from sour skim milk.

• *Sapsago:* This cheese, too, is made from soured skim milk with buttermilk added. It is light green in color and very hard and pungent, which makes it a perfect substitute for Parmesan. Although it contains only about 2 grams of fat per ounce, this same amount contains a high 520 milligrams of sodium. Because of its pungent taste, a little goes a long way.

Sapsago comes from Switzerland. But it is also made in Germany where it is called Glarnekase, Grunerkase, Schabziger, or Krauterkase.

• *Whip whipped cream with yogurt:* Instead of using whipped cream or the commercial toppings, both of which are high in cholesterol and/or saturated fats, use yogurt or tofu to top your desserts.

• *Switch from butter to margarine:* One tablespoon of butter has 30 milligrams of cholesterol, while an equal amount of margarine has 0 milligrams of cholesterol—once again, a small trade-off for a big reduction in cholesterol.

• *And make it tub margarine:* Solid margarines are high in hydrogenated vegetable oils, which have much the same reaction in the body as saturated fat does. Soft tub margarines made from corn, safflower, or sunflower oil are your best choice.

• *Spray and sprinkle popcorn:* Instead of buttering popcorn, spray it lightly with a nonstick vegetable coating and then sprinkle it with chili powder, onion powder, or cinnamon.

• *Spray those pans, too:* When you must sauté or fry foods, use one of the nonstick vegetable coatings instead of butter or margarine. They do the job of keeping food from sticking to pans, and they cut down on the oil in your diet without having much effect on taste.

• *Buy lean and go leaner:* Buy lean grades of meat and then trim visible fat.

• *Then broil, bake, or roast it:* Pan-fried meat retains its own fat while deep-fried meat becomes fatter from the oil it is cooked in. Broiled, baked, or roasted meat loses much of its fat in the cooking process. Worried about it drying out? Baste it with wine, tomato juice, or broth (but not with its own fat).

• *Then eat less of it:* Eat smaller amounts of meat or do as the Chinese do and mix small amounts of it with vegetables.

• *Feast on fins and feathers:* Lean beef has about twice the saturated fat of an equal amount of chicken breast. A fin fish like salmon has less saturated fat than chicken and much less cholesterol.

• *Make your own breading:* If you plan to have breaded meats, make your own breadings from plain bread crumbs. You can get these to stick to the meat by first dipping the meat in a mixture of skim milk and egg whites. Commercial breadings or prebreaded meats such as packaged chicken or fish sticks tend to be high in sodium and saturated fats.

• *Reach for low-fat items:* The food industry is responding to the public's demand for low-fat/low-cholesterol food items. These days there are low-fat sandwich meats, hot dogs, salad dressings, ice creams, and cheeses. Virtually everything that had a significant amount of fat in it is now available in a reduced-fat version.

Of course I recommend that you use these products in place of their high-fat cousins. Just remember to read the label to be sure they don't contain saturated fats. Low-fat is fine, but not if the remaining fat is saturated.

There is another catch to low-fat foods. They are usually made to replace a high-fat food, such as ice cream or bologna. Although the "low-fat" version certainly contains less fat than the food it is supposed to replace, it might still be high in fat.

To avoid fooling yourself, become a label reader.

• *Watch for these words on the labels:* Eggs, egg-yolk solids, whole milk, whole-milk solids, coconut, palm or palm-kernel oils, milk chocolate, imitation chocolate, lard, butter, hydrogenated or hardened oils, suet and animal byproducts. If the labels contain these items, the products contain saturated fat and should be left on the grocery shelf, or eaten infrequently and in limited amounts.

• *And really read the label:* And by reading the label I don't mean reading the front of the package where it may say "no cholesterol" or "all vegetable shortenings." Read the actual list of ingredients, searching for the items listed above.

Sometimes even that can be confusing. These statements sometimes list alternative sources of oil such as "soybean," "palm-kernel," and/or "cottonseed and coconut oils." There is no way for you to know which of the oils were used. In that situation, find a similar product that labels its ingredients more clearly.

Labels also list ingredients in decreasing order by weight. For example, cookies that have "palm-kernel oil" listed as the third ingredient on the label have much more saturated fat in them than cookies that list the same oil as the sixth ingredient.

UNSATURATED GOALS: 20 Percent or More

Unsaturated fats help reduce levels of serum cholesterol, too. That is why a goal of 20 percent or more is recommended.

Though the expert panel of the National Cholesterol Education Program recommends that we all reduce our consumption of saturated fats, they also recommend that our level of *polyunsaturated* fat consumption be *increased* from its current level of 5 percent to no more than 10 percent. (The panel recommends that polyunsaturated fats be limited to 10 percent because they are high in calories and because research is incomplete on the long-term effects of consuming more than that amount.)

The value of a polyunsaturated diet was discovered more than thirty years ago. It used to be thought that all fats reacted the same in the body. Then in 1952, Dr. J. Groen, working at the Wilhelmina Hospital in Amsterdam, revealed that when unsaturated fats replaced the saturated ones, cholesterol levels reversed.

To prove this, he tested three diets: vegetarian fare that allowed no butter or cream, a "frugal" European diet that was low in the saturated fat of animal products, and an "average" American diet high in saturated fats and cholesterol.

As you might expect, the diet high in unsaturated fats resulted in a low blood-cholesterol count, whereas the diet high in saturated fats resulted in a high blood-cholesterol count. The "frugal" diet fell in the middle.

To test his findings, Groen had the subjects switch diets. Their blood-cholesterol levels changed with the diets they were on, falling with the vegetarian diet and increasing with the saturated-fat diet. Since then this study has been repeated many times in many forms, always with the same results.

Monos vs. LDLs

Monounsaturates, according to the panel, should comprise 10 to 15 percent of your total calories. These fatty acids, found mainly in olive oil, sunflower-seed oil, safflower oil, and canola oil, react differently in the body from the polys.

Where polyunsaturates lower total cholesterol in the bloodstream, monounsaturates focus their attentions only on the bad guys, LDLs.

This was shown in research by Scott Grundy at the University of Texas, Dallas, and Fred Mattson at the University of California, San Diego. They fed subjects diets high in polyunsaturates and diets high in monounsaturates. Although both lowered cholesterol, the monos reduced LDLs only, leaving the HDLs free to do their job of cleaning the bloodstream.

Perhaps that is why University of Minnesota researcher Ancel Keyes found such low incidence of heart disease in the Mediterranean where diets are rich in olive oil. His examination of diets in seven countries showed that men in that region had less than half the chance of developing heart disease as did American men. Although

they ate less total fat and cholesterol than Americans, these Mediter-
raneans also had monounsaturates going for them.

Table 5 shows the common sources of unsaturated fats and their fat
breakdown per tablespoon. As you can see, all of these foods contain
saturated fat, but in amounts below the poly- and mono-unsaturated
fats.

Table 5. COMMON SOURCES OF UNSATURATED FATS

	Poly- (g)	Mono- (g)	Saturated (g)
Polyunsaturated Oils			
Safflower oil	10.1	1.6	1.2
Sunflower oil	8.9	2.7	1.4
Corn oil	8.0	3.3	1.7
Soybean oil	7.9	3.2	2.0
Monounsaturated Oils			
Canola oil	4.5	8.7	0.8
Peanut oil	4.3	6.2	2.3
Olive oil	1.1	9.9	1.8
Margarines			
Safflower oil (tub)	6.3	3.3	1.2
Corn oil (tub)	4.5	4.5	2.1
Corn oil (stick)	3.3	5.4	2.1
Soybean oil (tub)	3.9	5.1	1.8
Soybean oil (stick)	3.6	5.4	1.8
Nuts			
Walnuts	2.9	1.0	0.3
Brazil nuts	2.1	2.0	1.4
Peanuts	1.4	2.2	0.6
Pecans	1.1	2.8	0.4
Almonds	1.0	3.0	0.4
Cashews	0.7	2.3	0.8
Pistachio	0.6	2.6	0.5
Macadamia	0.1	4.9	0.9
Seeds			
Sunflower	2.9	0.9	0.5
Sesame	2.0	0.6	1.7
Pumpkin	1.8	0.7	1.2
Shortenings			
Cottonseed	3.3	5.7	3.2
Soybean	3.3	5.7	3.2

Sinister Sodium

Sodium is a necessary element for life. It helps regulate blood pressure, is necessary for nerve transmission, and is involved in the metabolism of protein and carbohydrates. On the whole you need about 1,100 to 3,300 milligrams daily. But the average American takes in about 5,000 milligrams per day, an overload that is easy to reach when you consider that a mere teaspoon of salt contains about 2,000 milligrams of sodium.

Unlike cholesterol, excess salt in your diet is not always easy to detect. Many people eat large amounts of salt and sodium and show no adverse response. Others eat much less of them than the normal population and still have high blood pressure.

Still, sodium levels should be kept within the low range. Sodium serves to retain fluid in fat cells, which are capable of expanding to eight times their size. This additional weight—called water weight—provides an extra burden for the body, the heart in particular. There is good evidence, furthermore, that too much salt for too long a period of time might lead to a kidney malfunction that forces the blood pressure higher.

High blood pressure—indeed even salt itself—has been shown to speed the development of atherosclerosis. Not only does the increased pressure contribute to the deposition of plaque, but too much sodium also causes the smooth muscle cells in the artery to contract and become stiff and enlarged. The larger these artery muscles become, the smaller the lumen, the area for blood flow through the artery.

If you reduce the amount of sodium in your body, these smooth muscle cells have the opportunity to "relax" to a smaller size. This reduction in the size of the smooth muscles serves to make the artery larger.

Maintaining a low-sodium diet, especially for someone who already has high blood pressure, is a difficult task. For instance, a McDonald's milk shake has a sodium content higher than that of a McDonald's Quarter Pounder. Sodium is in virtually everything we eat and drink, but some foods contain much more than others. It is added in salad dressings, canned vegetables, soups, and almost every precooked and processed food found in the supermarket. It is even found in ALKA-SELTZER, sugar-free soft drinks, and penicillin.

Foods such as potato chips, regular luncheon meats and hot dogs, bacon, and canned ham are so loaded with sodium that one meal's worth can provide much more than the maximum recommended daily amount. In fact, it is shocking to find that the diet foods of some major food manufacturers are so loaded with sodium that they can't be recommended to patients. The same is true of some low-sodium soups. Although they are lower in sodium than the regular variety, they are still too high to fit comfortably into the goals of the reversal diet program.

There are some keys to lowering sodium in the diet that you can undertake on your own. The first one is probably obvious—avoid the salt shaker. Another way is to follow this advice:

• *Avoid processed foods:* "Eat fresh" whenever you can. It is the rare processed food that doesn't contain added sodium as a preservative and a flavoring agent. Especially avoid foods that use sodium or salt as their main preserving agent, such as salted herring or salted beef. In Newfoundland, where salt intake is high from a diet of salted fish and meats, high blood pressure and strokes are three times more prevalent than in other Canadian provinces. The alarming intake of 25 or more grams of salt is equally disastrous.

Processing adds sodium to the most ordinary of foods. For instance, 100 grams of fresh green beans have 100 mg of sodium. The same amount of canned green beans has 236. Fresh carrots have 50 mg per 100 grams, canned have 236.

Read labels to see if salt and sodium have been added. If so, avoid those products.

• *Substitute salt:* The most "abused" form of sodium is ordinary table salt. Avoid using it by substituting flavors such as cayenne, cinnamon, clover, curry powder, dill, garlic powder, lime or lemon juice, nutmeg, onion powder, oregano, pepper, paprika, thyme, and vinegar.

Condiments such as soy sauce, mustard, ketchup, and Worcestershire sauce are also loaded with sodium. Salt free versions of these products provide the same taste *without* the sodium.

• *Eat more fruit:* Potassium, which is abundant in fruit, is known to lower blood pressure and serves to negate some of the ill-effects of sodium. Vegetarians who have a high potassium intake have a tendency toward normal blood pressure. And rural South Americans who consume plant ashes, which are high in potassium, as part of their diet have lower blood pressure than urban South Americans who have a diet high in sodium.

Potassium is necessary for normal heart function. Deficiencies can lead to heartbeat irregularities and serious heart-muscle damage.

The recommended daily intake of potassium for adults is 1,875 to 5,625 milligrams but in contrast to its counterpart sodium, it is difficult to get too much.

Table 6 gives some excellent sources of potassium.

Table 6. SOURCES OF POTASSIUM	
Food	Potassium (mg)
Cantaloupe, ½	880
Tomato	690
Banana	630
Baked potato	590
Strawberries, 2 cups	540
Squash, summer, 1 cup	510
Apricots, 3 dried	500
Squash, winter, ½ cup	450
Cauliflower, 1 cup	400
Watermelon, ½ slice	380
Corn, 1 ear	365
Orange	360
Turkey (fresh), 4 oz	350
Spinach, ½ cup	295
Hamburger, lean, 3 oz	290

Making Good Change

TRICKS FOR GETTING THE LEAD OUT

Knowing how to get rid of saturated fats, cholesterol, and sodium is one thing: *doing* it is another. A psychological approach is needed in making any change in habit that is as ingrained as our eating patterns.

I'll offer some simple psychological tricks for staying on an artery-clearing diet. But first let's take a look at how one individual, Dr. William Castelli, made changes in his diet.

Dr. Castelli, the current director of the Framingham Study, has been examining heart disease and its risk factors for many years and knows the "numbers" of heart disease as well as anyone. But one day Castelli realized that his own numbers were against him. His father, a physician, had had a heart attack before the age of fifty and had had his leg amputated from atherosclerosis when he was fifty-two. His mother died of a stroke when she was sixty-two. And now his brother was having angina attacks and he was only in his early forties.

Castelli measured his own serum-cholesterol level and found it to be an alarming 270. He realized that his cholesterol was 30 to 40 points higher than that of many people in his own study who were dying of heart attacks! He knew he needed to change his vital numbers. He took his research home and discussed it with his family. Their decision? They decided to make slow and steady changes.

They continued to eat beef, but in smaller portions. Extra money went to buy extra-lean cuts. They switched from whole milk to low-fat. Margarine came "in" and butter went "out." Hot dogs, bacon, and salami have been replaced by fish and chicken. Ice cream has gone the way of egg yolks in the Castelli residence.

As a result of these slow and steady changes Dr. Castelli has reduced his serum cholesterol by 60 points. He improved his numbers even further because of regular exercise.

Castelli's attitude has changed so much that sometimes he even orders fried eggs with no yolks when he's in a restaurant. "Why not?" he declares. "The menu specifically says 'eggs any style.'"

• *First tip: Make changes slowly:* Castelli changed his diet the right way. He didn't make radical changes that he might not have been able to maintain. Instead, he recognized problem areas and whittled away at them at a slow and steady pace.

There are many other psychological tricks to making good changes that I have taught and been taught over the years. All of them won't have significance for you. Some will seem downright mundane. Choose the ones that you think you can actually follow through on.

Let's start with tips for everyday living:

• *Think of this effort as an adventure:* Rather than feeling deprived of certain foods, think instead of the pleasure you can derive from trying new and different things to eat. Most of us eat the same ten meals all of our lives. This is an opportunity to taste a whole new world.

Look at some of the satisfying fare that can be substituted for high-fat, high-cholesterol foods and the calories they can save:

- 1 slice of angel-food cake instead of devil's-food avoids 8 grams of fat and 41 mg of cholesterol.
- 1 cup of plain popcorn instead of 1 ounce of potato chips avoids 4 grams of saturated fat.
- 1 cup of 1 percent low-fat milk instead of 1 cup of whole milk saves 8 grams of fat and 23 mg of cholesterol.
- A bagel instead of a Danish pastry saves 10 grams of fat and almost 50 mg of cholesterol.
- 1 baked potato instead of ½ cup home-fried potatoes saves 8 grams of fat.

These satisfying substitutes offer fewer calories and contain less fat which—as you know—can cloud your blood with fat globules and cholesterol. Simple changes like these will make a visible change in your waistline as well as the invisible change of reversing heart disease.

• *Snack before going to parties:* An apple, diet soda, or even water will appease the nervous appetite that you sometimes take to a party which otherwise can lead you to the saturated-fat snacks that abound there.

• *Don't feel beholden:* If you are served foods high in saturated fat or cholesterol, don't feel as though you have to eat them. And don't feel as though you have to comment when the waiter or hostess takes away your plate. There is no reason to be self-conscious about healthy living.

• *Don't bake holiday treats for friends:* Instead, give the treats that you receive to friends and keep the heart-healthy treats that you make for yourself. Or, if you feel guilty in doing that, discard them and share the heart-healthy treats that you make for yourself. That way, you know for sure what is in those Christmas goodies.

• *At home, control the menu:* Don't think you have to serve high-fat foods to please your family or friends. Most people are intrigued by meals that make them healthier.

• *Limit alcohol intake:* Extra calories aside, alcohol can lower your resistance to temptation. The less alcohol you drink, the less likely you are to stray from a planned diet.

TO AVOID OVEREATING:

• *Slow down, chew with purpose:* Take at least twenty minutes to consume a meal. Taking longer to eat will make you feel as though you are eating more. Besides, as heart researcher Irvine Page said, "Eat slowly because you will not eat as much and you might find time to say something between bites. Dining was meant to be for conversation and companionship, not nourishment alone."

• *Eat only while sitting down:* Much extra food is consumed on the run. Making it a point to sit down while eating will help you think about how much you are consuming.

• *Eat off of smaller plates:* Smaller plates create the impression that they are loaded with food.

• *Drink a 12-ounce glass of water before eating:* Water before a meal will take up room in your stomach, making you less hungry.

• *Never skip a meal:* Skipping meals lowers your blood sugar and makes you more hungry when the next meal comes around. Eat three healthy meals a day.

• *Wait ten minutes before snacking:* Between-meal snacks are usually impulsive acts. A wait before eating them will often make you realize you aren't hungry after all.

• *Keep the right stuff up front:* Make foods such as fruit and vegetables readily available by keeping them in the front of the refrigerator shelves.

If you follow the advice in this chapter, your cholesterol level is likely to drop and maybe even plummet. Other things will certainly happen, too, including weight loss and a dramatic increase in energy.

Although it may be a struggle to make these changes at first, they will become a natural part of your life-style in a very short period of time. It usually isn't long before the patients with whom I have shared this advice are looked upon admiringly by their friends, who most often decide that they too want to change their diets.

DEFENSIVE EATING

*The
"F" Words:
Fins and
Fiber*

5

D r. Denis Burkitt is an expert on stools—not the kind you sit on, but the kind you produce.

This charming Englishman spent many years in Africa where he made some astute observations on cardiovascular health based upon the stools that Africans left on the side of the road. He noticed that the "works" of the Africans were large and firm, in contrast to those of Western people (like himself) who had small, runny ones.

Since Africans have less coronary artery disease than Westerners, Burkitt did research in the 1960s to find out if their fiber-filled diets served to lower cholesterol.

His conclusion: *A fiber-rich diet speeds the transit of food through the body, reducing cholesterol absorption.*

His findings led to Burkitt's rules of diet: "Double the fiber, double the starch, reduce fat by half, reduce sugar by half, only eat whole grain breads, and give your frying pan to your neighbor."

Fiber is also in common laxatives containing psyllium, (Metamucil or its generic equivalent), found on the grocery shelf.

In Oregon, M. René Malinow was researching the reversal of heart disease in primates. He fed saponin, a substance derived from alfalfa, to animals with atherosclerosis. Though they remained on a high-fat, high-cholesterol diet their blockages decreased or stopped growing. Malinow had confirmed that in addition to the effects of the fiber in alfalfa, the saponin also had a unique effect of binding directly to cholesterol. In contrast, fiber lowers cholesterol by shortening the transit time of food through the intestinal tract and "sticks" to cho-lesterol containing bile which then passes out of the body through the stools. In addition, bile sequestrants (colestipol and cholestyramine) adsorb and combine with the bile acid in the intestine to form an insoluble complex which is excreted in the stool. This results in a partial removal of bile acids and prevents their reabsorption.

Malinow has conducted several regression experiments on monkeys which are fed a high-cholesterol diet to produce atherosclerosis. These lesions are then reversed by adding saponin, bile sequestrants, or combinations to the same cholesterol-rich diet that caused the lesions: The saponin binds directly to cholesterol, the bile sequestrants bind to bile acids, and the fiber shortens the transit time through the intestinal tract.

In humans as well bile sequestrants help reverse heart disease and the chances of developing heart disease.

In a 1984 study conducted by the National Heart, Lung and Blood Institute atherosclerosis was reversed in some members of a group of 1,800 people with heart disease. They were treated with diet modifications and bile-sequestrant fibers and given arteriograms at the beginning of the study and 7.4 years later when the study ended. The result was a reduction in the size of some of the blockages and a great reduction in the incidences of heart attacks.

Variations on this same study have been repeated many times with similar results: Fiber, especially water-soluble fiber, reduces cholesterol levels.

Proving Fiber

Many studies have shown that high-fiber diets are responsible for lower cholesterol levels and lower rates of heart disease. One recently concluded study of Chinese eating habits by T. Colin Campbell, a Cornell University nutritional biochemist, credited their high-fiber diet and the fact that they eat less meat and dairy products with a national average serum cholesterol of 127 mg/dl—85 points lower than the American average. The study shows that the Chinese eat at least 34 grams of fiber a day compared to the American average of 11 grams.

A similar story came from a study of autopsies on 150 Japanese civilians living in Okinawa made by U.S. Army Dr. P. E. Steiner. He was able to find only seven cases of atherosclerosis, none of them severe. In 150 American autopsies, we would find that roughly half of autopsies of males over the age of forty would show signs of atherosclerosis. Steiner reported the Japanese to be "amazingly free of degenerative diseases of the cardiovascular system." He credited their low-cholesterol levels to their diet, which consists of little meat and a lot of rice, sweet potatoes, soybeans, and vegetables.

And in Africa, where dietary fiber can exceed 150 grams a day in some ethnic groups, Dr. H. C. Trowel of Uganda performed 6,500 autopsies on members of the Bantu group from 1930 to 1956 and reported in the British medical journal *The Lancet* that he was unable to find a single case of heart disease. "Coronary heart disease [among the Bantu] is almost non-existent," he said.

Of course, to be as healthy as a Bantu, you would have to live like a Bantu, which in our society of convenience foods, is mighty tough to do. Maybe instead we should live a little more like the Chinese. They eat about three times the amount of fiber we do on a given day. And they eat about 20 percent more calories, too, simply because theirs is a plant-based diet instead of one based on meat and dairy foods like ours.

Since the fat in your diet is more easily digested, it sticks to your ribs—and your stomach and thighs. The fat in a plant-based diet is tough for your body to use. First your body has to work harder to extract it from the undigestible fiber. Second, your body has less time to absorb fat before food passes through the bowel in this fibrous version of a rapid transit system. Finally, there isn't as much fat in a plant-based diet, which is why you rarely see overweight Chinese in their home country. They eat rice, grain, fruit, vegetables, occasionally fish, and on major holidays, a duck or pig if they can afford it. Their cholesterol goes from 160 at age sixteen to about 180 at age eighty, and they are one-sixth as likely to die of heart disease as Americans their same age.

The same is true of other national diets, as Dr. Jeremiah Stamler and his associates have discovered. They examined the content of fiber, sugar, and dietary lipids in the national diet of twenty countries and found that a high consumption of fiber relates to low rates of heart disease. The key reason for this reduction, the investigators believed, was the lower serum cholesterol of those on the high-fiber diets.

The Oat-Bran Boom

But in it was a study carried out by Dr. James Anderson, a professor of medicine and nutrition at the University of Kentucky, that really got America interested in oat bran.

He fed ten people 100 grams of oat bran a day for twenty-one days and achieved a 19 percent reduction in cholesterol levels. Although his work essentially repeated that of many other researchers, it came at a time of heightened concern about cholesterol and questions about how to reduce it easily.

In the spring of 1988, the *Journal of the American Medical Association* concluded that oat bran was the least expensive method for reducing cholesterol.

After that report, oat bran took off. The oat-bran muffin became the croissant of the eighties. Every bakery worth its flour now sells a variety of oat-bran muffins, including raisin, cranberry, and chocolate chip (not on the list of reversal foods, I hasten to add).

Oat bran itself has become so popular that food manufacturers have been forced to import oats from as far away as Poland and Argentina to manufacture such delicacies as cereals, bagels, tortilla chips, and even ice-cream toppings. Recently, a study in the *New England Journal of Medicine* showed that much of the "magic" of oat bran was due simply to the fact that it replaces foods that are higher in saturated fat. Although oat bran definitely binds with bile to pass it from the body, the current study reached similar conclusions to those of Dr. Burkitt: starchy carbohydrates—including oat bran—are healthy fare, especially when eaten in place of foods with saturated fats.

According to Dr. William Connor, quoted from an editorial on fiber in the *New England Journal of Medicine:* "Clearly, people who eat large quantities of oat bran or other, similar cereals for breakfast have little room for bacon and eggs, and that may be all to the good."

Is this oat-bran mania justified? I think it's great. It introduces the nation to a heart-healthy food that wasn't given a second glance by most people a few years ago. It gets people accustomed to new tastes and new ways of cooking. It might even make them think about eating other foods in this cholesterol-lowering category known as soluble fibers.

To quote Dr. Connor again: "One could use a variety of starchy carbohydrates, such as rice, potatoes, pasta, bread, beans, any one of many cereal products, including oat bran, and fruits and vegetables—all of which would provide the wide range of choices necessary in any program of dietary change."

The Soluble Solution

Oat bran is only one of dozens of foods known as soluble fibers. That means simply that the fibers in these types of food dissolve in water to form a jellylike substance that binds cholesterol and bile acids (which are synthesized from cholesterol) and keeps them from being absorbed into the bloodstream.

In one important study conducted by David Blankenhorn at USC, eighty men were given bile sequestrants, the B vitamin niacin, and a target diet of no more than 125 mg of cholesterol per day. A second group of eighty-two men was given a placebo and a target diet that included 250 mg of cholesterol per day. All of the men had had coronary-bypass surgery prior to the study.

Of the group treated with bile sequestrants, 61 percent of the patients showed no increase in the size of the blockage in their arteries two years after surgery. Better news was that 16 percent showed a reversal of clogging in their coronary arteries. Of the group given only dietary intervention, 39 percent showed no change in the size of their blockages while 2.4 percent showed a reversal in the clogging of their coronary arteries.

This study is a prime example of the effect bile sequestrants have on heart disease.

If you are keen on taking laxatives as a quick way of increasing soluble fiber in your diet, 3 teaspoons of psyllium (contained in Metamucil) added to a daily glass of juice have been shown to lower blood cholesterol by as much as 15 percent. Psyllium are certainly one of the cheaper sources of soluble fiber. The only known side-effects are increased bowel movements and a period of gassiness.

REAL FOOD FIBER

If you feel more comfortable getting soluble fiber from "real" food, there are plenty of sources available.

You could try to use oat bran exclusively, as Anderson's study group did. But to experience the extraordinary reduction in cholesterol of his group requires an extraordinary consumption of oat bran, about 100 grams per day. In "dry" terms, that equals about two-thirds of a cup of oat bran. In muffin terms, that could translate into as many as ten oat-bran muffins per day, depending upon the amount of oat bran used in baking the muffin.

What is more, all commercially produced muffins are not created equal, as a 1989 *New York Times* study of the muffin market proved. The *Times* analyzed fifty muffins from thirty bakeries around the country for their nutritional content. The results were shocking in their disparity. Some contained so little oat bran that they were almost worthless as a source of fiber. A couple contained so much fat (29 grams) that they equaled three small bags of potato chips in fat content. To get 100 grams of oat bran from the muffins of one of the large bakeries analyzed, more than fourteen muffins would have to be consumed. Along with that humanly impossible feat would come 5,190 calories, 100 grams of fat, and 6,006 milligrams of sodium—definitely not an example of a reversal diet.

With the specter of that much daily oat-bran consumption, it is nice to know about the other foods that make up soluble fiber. These fall under the categories of pectins (found in almost all fruits and some vegetables) and gums (found in oat bran and beans).

MEAT ANALOGUES AS REVERSAL FOODS

Meat analogues are products that contain no meat or animal fat and rely instead upon a combination of vegetables, grains, and spices to approximate the taste and consistency of meat. I include them in this section because they are usually made of soluble fibers that have no saturated fats and serve to lower cholesterol levels.

There are several of these meatless "meats" on the market. One of the better ones is Vege-Burger, made by Loma Linda foods. Right out of the can, it has the consistency of cooked ground beef and can be mixed with egg whites, bread crumbs, spices, and onion to make meatballs or "vege-burger" patties that serve as excellent substitutes for "real" hamburger.

Also included in the recipe section of this book are several cholesterol-free vegetarian recipes aimed at providing an alternative to meat.

If you are feeling adventurous you might try some of these. Not only do they have excellent flavor, but they are also made with soluble fibers such as lentils and soy beans and contain no cholesterol or saturated fat. They are the perfect reversal foods and can help satisfy the craving for meat that so many of us carnivores have.

Don't Shun Insolubles

Fibers that don't dissolve in water are called insolubles. Technically, these fibers fall into three categories: cellulose, lignin, and hemicellulose. They haven't received as much publicity as their soluble kin have, but as we know from the work of Burkitt and other researchers, insoluble fibers are also effective in reducing cholesterol levels.

This is the type of fiber you may know as roughage because it can't be broken down by the body's digestive juices. But in reality it functions as "softage" because it creates soft and easily passed stools. Although insolubles can't be broken down, they do absorb water like a sponge, increasing in size many times once they get into the bowel.

It's this increase in size that speeds the transit time of food through the body and soaks up cholesterol-carrying bile acids on the way. Quite simply, the digested food of a fiber eater has to leave more quickly to make room for more food. That is one reason why Africans, Japanese, Chinese, and vegetarians have more frequent bowel movements and less frequent heart disease.

But those who eat low-fiber diets (as most Americans do) have digested food in their bowel that can compress and make more room for incoming food without having to leave the body. This leads to less frequent bowel movements and allows the cholesterol to stay in the bowel longer and be reabsorbed into the bloodstream.

Lower Blood Pressure

But lower cholesterol levels aren't the only reason for you to consume a lot of fiber. Added bulk in the diet has been shown to lower blood pressure as well. The generally accepted reason for this is that fibrous foods contain less sodium and more potassium. This combination has been shown to lower blood pressure in many people. That is why vegetarian groups such as the Seventh Day Adventists and some Mormon communities have much lower blood pressure than the rest of the American population. They don't drink alcohol or smoke cigarettes, they avoid salt, they have a potassium intake of about 5,000 to 6,000 milligrams which they get from the 50 grams of fiber they eat every day!

FIBER RECOMMENDATION: 35 Grams a Day

If you consume the typical American diet, you will most likely have to increase the amount of fiber in your meals to realize its cholesterol-lowering value. On the average we Americans consume about 11 grams of fiber per day. But many whose diet is largely limited to fast food (and you know who you are) take in almost no fiber at all.

As heart-healthy advice, I recommend a daily consumption of at least 35 grams of fiber. More fiber than that won't hurt, by any means. In fact I think it's virtually impossible to get too much fiber in your diet, since a variety of fibrous foods contain all the nutrients the human body needs.

But I recommend 35 grams a day to start for two reasons:

• **It doesn't interfere greatly with normal eating patterns:** It is possible to increase fiber intake greatly by replacing or adding a few foods in your normal daily diet. An apple a day, for instance, adds about 4 grams of fiber as does a baked potato or a serving of kidney beans. And Dr. Denis Burkitt recommends substituting whole-wheat bread for white bread. That simple change alone can add several grams of fiber each day, depending upon how much the flour has been refined.

You can easily add these beneficial foods without making abrupt changes in diet that would be difficult to adhere to.

• **It has shown significant results:** As explained in this chapter, a diet containing about 35 grams of fiber has been shown to make a significant impact on the cholesterol levels, blood pressure, and the other vital numbers that reverse chances of heart disease.

Dr. Anderson and his fellow researchers at the University of Kentucky say that cholesterol levels can be reduced about 20 percent by eating a diet with 20 to 35 grams of total fiber a day of which 7 to 12 grams are soluble. As a source of soluble fiber he recommends oat bran, oatmeal and corn, and legumes such as pinto beans, lentils, and peas.

There are several ways to tell if you are getting enough fiber in your diet. The most obvious way is by weighing food and counting the number of grams, using the food chart provided at the end of this section. I recommend that approach in the beginning just to discover your baseline fiber intake. You'll be keeping a daily diet anyway as part of the reversal diet program, so recording fiber won't be much extra effort.

Later on, when the reversal diet becomes a part of your life-style, there will be an easier way to tell if you are getting enough fiber. The bulky, rapid-transit nature of fiber increases the number and ease of your bowel movements. If you are eating 35 grams of fiber a day, you can expect to be having two or three bowel movements a day. Transit time should decrease from the two to five days that is average for Americans to twelve to twenty-four hours, which is average for fiber eaters. The higher the fiber intake, the faster the transit time.

If you are curious enough, you can test your own transit time by eating some beets. They maintain their red color even after they are passed.

Increased dietary fiber and faster transit time have benefits besides those for the heart. They have been linked directly to lower rates of colon cancer, gallstones, obesity, varicose veins, and hemorrhoids. The reasons for this aren't totally clear, but researchers like Burkitt speculate that low-fiber diets create a breeding ground for bacteria. These bacteria act like a carcinogen when they are in contact with the intestinal lining. A diet high in fiber isn't as good a breeding ground for bacteria. And since fiber speeds through the intestines, the bacteria it produces have much less contact with the intestinal lining.

There are short-term benefits of fiber, too. You will feel lighter and more energetic on a high-fiber diet. Fiber makes you as strong as a bull, because you are eating what the bull eats and not the bull itself.

Table 7.   GREAT FIBER SOURCES

Food	Amount	Fiber (g)
BREAD		
Country oat	2 slices	6.0
Whole-wheat, stone ground	2 slices	4.5
Wheat, reduced-calorie	2 slices	4.0
Mixed grain	2 slices	3.2
Rye	2 slices	3.1
English muffin, wheat	1 muffin	3.0
Pita, whole-wheat	1 pocket	2.8
Corn bread, whole ground	1 piece	2.7
Cracked wheat	2 slices	2.6
Bran muffin	1 muffin	2.5
Bran oat cakes	2 cakes	2.0
BREAKFAST CEREALS, COLD		
100% bran-type with added fiber	½ cup	14.0
100% bran-type	⅓ cup	10.0
100% bran-type with oat bran	½ cup	8.0

Food	Amount	Fiber (g)
Multibran	⅓ cup	6.5
Oatmeal flakes	1 cup	6.0
Corn bran, ready-to-eat	⅔ cup	5.4
40% bran-type flakes	⅔ cup	5.3
Bran-type flakes with raisins	1 oz	5.0
Oat bran, crunchy	1 oz	5.0
Bran squares	⅔ cup	4.6
BREAKFAST CEREALS, HOT		
Multibran, creamy, instant, dry	¼ cup	8.0
Oat bran	⅓ cup	5.0
Oatmeal, cooked	¾ cup	1.6
FRUIT		
Figs, dried	5	8.7
Pear	1 large	6.2
Blackberries	½ cup	4.5
Dates	5	3.2
Orange	1	3.1
Raspberries	½ cup	3.1
Prunes	5	3.0
Apple, with skin	1	3.0
Strawberries	¾ cup	2.9
Apricots, dried	10 halves	2.7
Kiwi	1	2.6
Nectarine	1	2.2
Cantaloupe	½ melon	2.0
Raisins	¼ cup	1.9
Banana	1	1.8
Plums	3 small	1.8
Blueberries	½ cup	1.7
Apricots	2	1.5
GRAINS		
Corn bran, raw	1 oz	23.0
Wheat bran, toasted	1 oz	14.1
Rice bran, raw	1 oz	6.2–9.5
Bulgur, raw	1 oz	5.2
Barley, raw	1 oz	4.9
Oat bran, raw	1 oz	4.3
Cornmeal, whole-grain	1 oz	4.3
Wheat flour, whole-grain	1 oz	3.6
Cornmeal, whole-grain	1 oz	3.1
Wheat germ	1 oz	3.0
Oats, rolled, dry	1 oz	2.9
Millet, hulled, raw	1 oz	2.4

Food	Amount	Fiber (g)
LEGUMES		
Baked beans, vegetarian, canned	½ cup	9.8
Kidney, cooked	½ cup	9.0
Pintos, cooked	½ cup	8.9
Black-eyed peas, cooked	½ cup	8.3
Miso (soybeans)	½ cup	7.5
Chick-peas	½ cup	7.0
Limas, cooked	½ cup	6.8
Navy, cooked	½ cup	6.8
Lentils, cooked	½ cup	5.2
White, cooked	½ cup	5.0
Green peas, cooked	½ cup	2.4
NUTS AND SEEDS		
Almonds, oil-roasted	¼ cup	4.4
Pistachio nuts	¼ cup	3.5
Mixed nuts, oil roasted	¼ cup	3.2
Peanuts	¼ cup	3.2
Pecans	¼ cup	2.3
RICE, PASTA, AND TORTILLAS		
Pasta, multigrain,		
with quinoa, dry	2 oz	8.0
with triticale, dry	2 oz	6.5
with oat bran, dry	2 oz	6.0
Whole-wheat, dry	2 oz	6.0
Rice, wild, cooked brown, long-grain, cooked	½ cup	5.3
Tortilla, corn	2 shells	3.1
SNACKS		
Crackers		
Stoned-wheat	1 oz	3.9
Crisps, thin oat	½ oz	3.2
Crisps, thin rye	½ oz	3.0
Hearty wheat	4 crackers	3.0
Whole-wheat saltines	5 crackers	1.0
Cookies		
Oat plus fruit	2 cookies	3.0
Graham crackers, oat bran	1.2 oz	3.0
Oat bran	2 cookies	2.8
Fig bars	2 cookies	1.3
Popcorn	½ oz	2.0
VEGETABLES		
Artichokes, raw	1 medium	6.7
Brussels sprouts, boiled	5 sprouts	4.5

Food	Amount	Fiber (g)
Mixed, frozen, cooked	½ cup	3.5
Sweet potato, baked	1 potato	3.4
Corn, cooked	1 ear	2.8
Parsley, chopped	1 cup	2.8
Parsnips, cooked	½ cup	2.7
Broccoli, raw, chopped	1 cup	2.5
Potato, with skin	1 medium	2.5
Carrots, raw	1 carrot	2.3
Turnip greens, boiled	½ cup	2.2
Spinach, boiled	½ cup	2.1
Asparagus, cut	1 cup	2.0
Cauliflower, cooked	5 florets	2.0
Zucchini, cooked	½ cup	1.8
Cabbage, raw, shredded	1 cup	1.8
Green beans, string, cooked	½ cup	1.6
Tomato, raw	1 medium	1.5

Source: "Soluble and Total Dietary Fiber in Selected Foods," and "Provisional Table on the Dietary Fiber Content of Selected Foods," USDA Human Nutrition Information Service.

The Friendly Fin

These days, if you see a fin swimming toward you, grab it if you are at the dinner table. Fish is good for your heart. So good, in fact, that a Dutch study showed that men who ate as little as seven ounces of fish a week were half as likely to die of heart disease over a twenty-year period as men who ate less than seven ounces. And two meals of fish per week have been shown to lower blood pressure substantially.

A group of European researchers proved this in a long-term study of eating habits of Dutch men. They watched the eating habits of 1,088 men in the town of Zutphen. After twenty years of analysis they were able to conclude that the risk of heart disease dropped as the consumption of fish went up. Here were their conclusions:

Table 8. FISH CONSUMPTION AND HEART DISEASE

Fish Eaten (pounds per year)	Incidence of Heart Disease	Fish Eaten (pounds per year)	Incidence of Heart Disease
0	Average	24–35	54% reduction
1–11	40% reduction	over 35	58% reduction
12–23	43% reduction		

The heart-helping part of the fish is called Omega-3 oil, a highly unsaturated fat that the fish get from the plankton they eat. This oil has a very low freezing point and functions as a sort of antifreeze in fish, keeping them from freezing in very cold water.

In humans, it has been shown to have some "anti-" properties, too:

• *It is anticholesterol:* In a small study conducted at the Oregon Health Sciences University the Omega-3 fatty acids have been shown to be two to five times more effective in reducing serum cholesterol than the Omega-6 fatty acids found in vegetable and seed oils. The fish-oil diet led to a substantial decrease in total cholesterol and an improvement in the HDL/total cholesterol ratio over a regular diet and a diet high in polyunsaturates.

• *It is antihypertensive:* Omega-3 fatty acids have been shown to lower blood pressure in fish eaters. In one of these studies, mackerel was eaten twice a week by a group of men with both normal and high blood pressure. The blood pressure of both of these groups dropped substantially while they ate the fish and went back up when their diet returned to normal.

• *It is an anticoagulant:* Omega-3 oil inhibits the body's production of prostaglandin, a chemical that inspires clotting.

As we know from Chapter 1, cholesterol and clots are important factors contributing to the buildup of atherosclerosis. Remove the factors and you can reverse or stop the buildup. Two important studies using Omega-3 oils have demonstrated just that.

A research team at the University of Texas Medical Center successfully prevented the recurrence of blockage in several heart-disease patients who had undergone balloon angioplasty, the opening of a blockage with a tiny balloon inserted into the coronary artery.

This procedure squashes the fatty plaque against the artery walls and improves circulation. But buildup often recurs again in about six months, a process known as "restenosis."

To avoid restenosis, a group of forty-three men with a total of fifty lesions opened with angioplasty were given a daily dose of Omega-3 fatty acids. The fish-oil treatment was started seven days before angioplasty and continued for six months after the procedure.

The results of the study, measured by coronary angiography, showed a return of some blockage in 8 of the 50 lesions (16 percent). In a group that didn't receive Omega-3 oil, there was a restenosis in

19 of 53 lesions (36 percent.) A similar study was conducted at George Washington University in Washington, D.C., with almost identical results. Quite simply, these studies show that fish oil prevents the buildup of atherosclerosis.

The anticoagulant effect of fish oil is the chief reason for this. Remember how cholesterol and clotted blood build up around damaged intima to form the atherosclerotic lesion? Omega-3 fatty acids greatly reduce the blood's ability to clot, which means that fibrinogen and red blood cells form more slowly—if at all—on a damaged artery.

Additional blockage prevention may also come from more Omega-3 oil seeping into the intima itself. The presence of this fatty acid in the intima makes the membrane less "reactive" and less likely to become inflamed, says Dr. Mark Milner, a professor of noninvasive cardiology at George Washington University.

These factors combined with the ability of this highly unsaturated fat to lower LDL cholesterol and produce a food with near-medicinal properties.

A LITTLE IS BETTER THAN A LOT

In fact, fish oil seems like such a wonder food that many people have begun taking it like a medicine, in fish-oil capsules they find in health-food stores. Although it can be prescribed like a medicine, it should be done so only by a doctor. Fish-oil capsules often contain far more vegetable oil than fish oil does. But even if you buy the ones that have high concentrations of fish oil, enormous amounts of extra calories can be picked up from these capsules of fat. And there is also a down side to fish oil. By consuming too much Omega-3 oil, you can increase your chances of stroke.

The possibility that a diet high in fish oil causes strokes was first noticed in Eskimos in Greenland, who eat an average of 325 pounds of fish per year (Americans eat less than 15). Although researchers found that the high concentration of Omega-3 fatty acids in their diet kept these generally obese people from having high cholesterol or many heart attacks, they also found that they were much more likely to have brain hemorrhages. Why? Though lower clotting factors might be good for the arteries of the heart, an excessively low amount can lead to increased bleeding, especially in the weaker, more vulnerable vessels of the brain.

FISH RECOMMENDATION:
TWO TO THREE MEALS A WEEK

That doesn't mean you should fear fish; you just shouldn't overdo it. It is great food, especially when eaten as a food and not taken as a capsule. In fact, here is what Dr. William Castelli, director of the Framingham Heart Study, says about our finned friends: "Fish should be put above everything else on the diet because it can actually reverse the process of arterial damage that leads to heart attacks."

How can you most safely take advantage of this wonder food without overdoing it? I think the medical studies provide a very clear answer: two or three meals a week of an oily, cold-water fish will greatly reduce your chance of heart disease and provide the effects necessary to reverse the buildup of blockage in the arteries.

Here are a few guidelines to maximize the benefits from your finned-fare:

• *Eat the oiliest fish:* Since Omega-3 oil functions as antifreeze, the highest concentration can be found in cold-water fish like king salmon, shad, lake sturgeon, and Atlantic mackerel. Approximately 10 to 15 percent of their body weight is Omega-3 oil.

Next highest, with 5 to 10 percent Omega-3 content, are salmon (coho, Atlantic, sockeye), trout (lake and rainbow), tuna (albacore, bluefin), bonito, herring, mackerel, whitefish, pompano, and carp.

Although other fish contain lower amounts of Omega-3 oils, eat them anyway. They still contain substantially more of this heart-healthy oil than other animal sources of protein, and they contain much less cholesterol and saturated fats.

• *Preparation counts:* Make sure you don't undo the benefits of eating fish by frying it in butter or breading it with a commercially prepared product that contains egg yolks, milk solids, or tropical oils. Keep preparation simple. Broil or grill the fish, flavoring or moistening it with olive oil, wine, or fruit juices like lemon or lime.

Also remember that deep-fried fish such as the type used in fast-food restaurants contain almost none of the beneficial oil and a lot of fat. If you see a fin from that kind of fish approaching, just let it pass you by.

OMEGA-3 SOURCES: FROM FISH TO NUTS

Table 9 lists foods rich in Omega-3 fatty acids.

Table 9. FOODS RICH IN OMEGA-3	
Foods	Omega-3 (g per 100 g of food)
SEAFOOD	
Atlantic Cod	0.23
Flounder	0.23
Halibut (Atlantic)	0.40
Halibut (Greenland)	0.51
Halibut (Pacific)	0.34
Herring (Atlantic)	0.92
Herring (Pacific)	1.36
Mackerel (Atlantic)	0.85
Rockfish	0.82
Salmon (Atlantic)	0.36
Salmon (Chinook)	1.83
Salmon (Coho)	1.80
Salmon (Sockeye)	3.31
Sole	0.18
Tuna (Canned Albacore)	0.52
Tuna (Canned Bluefin)	0.98
Clams	0.17
Crab (King)	0.52
Spiny lobster	0.28
Shrimp	0.34
VEGETABLE OILS	
Chestnut	4
Hempseed	19
Linseed	45
Perilla	67
Soybean	7
Walnut	4
Walnut, English	11
Wheat germ	7

. . . And More Defensive Foods

ALCOHOL AND GARLIC

Curious about the effects of alcohol on the rate of heart disease, Dr. Arthur Klatsky of Kaiser Permanente Hospital in Oakland, California, designed a study using the files of this massive institution. He and a team of researchers examined the medical histories of 120,000 patients and found that those who consumed an average of two alcoholic drinks a day were 40 percent less likely to be hospitalized for heart attacks than nondrinkers.

Curious about the results of Klatsky's study, researchers at Stanford University examined the blood of subjects who drank two and three drinks a day and found that they had higher levels of the good HDL cholesterol than nondrinking subjects. And although the type of cholesterol produced by alcohol is HDL-3 and not as high in quality as the HDL-2 variety found in people who exercise regularly, it is still the "good" cholesterol. Anyway you cut it, high levels of HDL mean lower risk of heart attack and a greater likelihood that arterial blockage is reversing.

Although Klatsky's findings have been confirmed many times, you shouldn't pour a third drink in toast of this fine researcher's work. Klatsky's other findings about alcohol have been confirmed, too: drinkers who averaged between three and five drinks per day had a 50 percent higher mortality rate than nondrinkers. Why? Two daily drinks appeared to have no effect upon blood pressure. But three or more per day caused a substantial rise in blood pressure. And six drinks per day doubled the chances of hypertension for white patients and increased it by 50 percent among blacks.

ALCOHOL RECOMMENDATIONS: TWO OUNCES PER DAY

There is no indication that one type of alcohol is better or worse than another. What is important is that you don't exceed about two ounces of alcohol per day. That equals a couple of beers, two small glasses of wine, or two small highballs. If you drink more than two ounces per day, I recommend reducing intake to that amount.

There is no reason to start drinking if you don't already just to pick up these extra HDLs. Although research shows us that they are there for the moderate drinker, I don't think you should start a potentially bad habit to get them.

AND FINALLY GARLIC

Garlic deserves mention here as a defensive food, although many people find that its lingering odor puts it in the category of an offensive food.

Garlic has been shown to reduce serum-cholesterol levels in both man and animal experiments. In one human experiment reported in *Artery*, twenty healthy adults were fed garlic oil for six months. Their total cholesterol dropped 16 percent whereas their HDL rose 40 percent.

The same researcher, A. Bordia, conducted a controlled trial on sixty-two heart-disease patients. After ten months of daily doses of garlic oil, there was a 23 percent drop in serum cholesterol.

The reason garlic hasn't caught on the way oat bran has is the amount of garlic required to achieve these results. In Bordia's experiments, the subjects were given 15 milligrams of garlic oil (equal to 30 grams of whole garlic). That is a lot of garlic to eat on a daily basis.

GARLIC RECOMMENDATIONS: EAT IT

Of course garlic isn't medicine, it's food. If you like it, keep using it. It may never replace the oat-bran muffin as a great breakfast, but it can certainly contribute a lot of flavor to a great meal.

ON
THE
ROAD

*Fast Food
or Gourmet, the
Reversal Diet
Can Travel*

6

D iets travel better than they used to, but they still don't travel very well. Leave the controlled environment of the home and you are surrounded by a world of culinary temptations.

It takes the strongest resolve to stick to a diet when dining out. And it isn't only an issue with fast-food restaurants. Fat is flavor in most foods. And the law of the jungle is that the restaurants with the most flavorful fare survive.

After forty-eight years as a heart researcher and preventive cardiologist, I am convinced that heart-healthy meals can be found in practically any restaurant, even if it takes a microscope and a creative mind to find them. Like Dr. Castelli, who found that "eggs any style" also meant those without yolks, people are learning to make demands on restaurants that are reshaping the way we eat. For instance, public comment on the lard-filled cooking oil that McDonald's used led the restaurant chain to switch to polyunsaturated vegetable oils in some of their products. And a desire for chicken meals that aren't deep-fried has led to an increase in fast-food restaurants that broil their fare.

This health awareness on the part of many restaurants and the public they serve has led to a definite decline in the amount of fat in our diets and a lowering of the average American's serum-cholesterol level. But relying on general trends in the food industry to put your numbers into the reversal range is an approach that isn't going to work. "Won't power" and preplanning are still necessary to avoid restaurant food that can ruin your reversal diet.

A Strategy for Fast Foods

A few years ago it would have been virtually impossible to recommend anything at a fast-food restaurant that would be in keeping with the reversal diet. There was no alternative to food fried in lard, "juicy" hamburgers that were dripping with fat and cholesterol, and milk shakes that were little more than cups of fat.

Fast-food restaurants are still dietary minefields. But fast-food outlets not only prepare food fast, they also respond quickly to the wants and needs of the public they serve. So a restaurant like Wendy's, which would have been off-limits to reversal dieters a few years ago, now has two exciting additions to the menu in their salad bar and baked potato. Eaten with the proper ingredients, these are ideal reversal foods.

McDonald's menu of nonreversal foods has been supplemented with a bevy of boxed salads that are excellent reversal meals if skimmed of the fatty meats and salad dressings that are included with some of them.

Salad bars are springing up in so many fast-food chains that some food-industry experts think they may be the major source of vegetables for many people. Indeed, since one-fifth of the American public eats fast food on any given day, that may well be true. That is good news, as is most anything that can be done to distract the public from artery-clogging choices.

But salad bars in fast-food outlets can still be nutritionally dangerous. Lurking beneath the salad greens is often a variety of high-fat, high-cholesterol condiments such as bacon bits, cheddar cheese, rich dressings, and potato salad and other goodies that can make your body wish you had eaten a double hamburger with cheese. Salad bars frequently contain such nonreversal foods as barbecued spareribs, boiled eggs, potato salad made with mayonnaise, a variety of fattening cheeses, and deep-fried items such as batter-dipped tofu. With "salad" like that, it would be easy to get your daily allotment of cholesterol and fat with just one meal.

To be on the reversal-diet program, you have to fill your plate with things that come from the ground and not with things that graze on top of it. That means to reach for miniature corn and kidney beans and skip eggs, cheese, and meats. A little meat might be fine, whereas a little more might not. There is good evidence that we Americans are eating more protein than we need and are suffering some ill effects. Remember, you are trying to keep meat consumption down to about six ounces to avoid saturated fat and cholesterol. And on a salad, garbanzos and kidney beans have a meaty flavor that might satisfy your carnivorous needs.

Opt for oil-and-vinegar dressing or nonfat, no-cholesterol dressings if available in place of fatty salad dressings such as Thousand Island

and Roquefort. Or try squeezing fresh lemon on your salad. Remember that many prepared salads are frequently made with fattening dressings such as mayonnaise, a product that contains large amounts of cholesterol and fat.

The difference between a reversal salad and a nonreversal one can be astonishing, as this nutritional breakdown of two salads shows:

Table 10.   SALADS—RIGHT AND WRONG

The Right Stuff Ingredient	Calories	Fat (g)	Sodium (mg)
3 leaves of lettuce	2	0	1
3½ oz garbanzo beans	180	2.4	50
1 oz bean sprouts	10	0	0
¼ red pepper	5	0	3
3 cauliflower flowerets	7	0	3
2 broccoli flowerets	7	0	3
1 miniature corn	18	0.1	0
1 carrot round	2	0	1
½ cup red cabbage	15	0	13
2 cherry tomatoes	10	0	1
1 tbsp oil & vinegar	50	5	0
Totals:	306	7.5	75
The Wrong Stuff Ingredient	Calories	Fat (g)	Sodium (mg)
Barbecued sparerib (5 oz)	125	8.0	400
1 egg	78	5.5	59
Carrot & raisin salad (5 oz)	198	20.0	100
½ oz cheddar cheese	55	4.5	100
1 oz batter-dipped tofu	100	10.0	4
8 strips of tempu	150	20.0	35
¼ cup potato salad	60	3.5	250
Totals:	766	71.5	948

Source: Gannett Westchester Newspapers, Nov. 30, 1988, p. E-1.

The same rule of thumb goes for baked potatoes. Don't douse them with chili or cheese sauce. Instead, order the potato plain and moisten it with margarine and nonfat milk. Add pepper and a touch of salt, and you have a fast and filling meal without cholesterol and with little fat.

Fast Foods Are Not Created Equal

Of course I can't pretend that salad bars and baked potatoes are the only things offered in fast-food restaurants. Fast-food menus are built around hamburgers, french fries, pizza, chicken, milk shakes, turnovers and so on.

For the most part fast foods—especially of the fried variety—should be passed over in the reversal diet. But in reality that is almost impossible for some people. Whether out of necessity or just mere convenience, many reversal dieters are going to find themselves stuck in a place where they can have only fast foods to rely upon. In that case you can make some careful choices to avoid consuming too much cholesterol.

Table 11. CHOLESTEROL IN FAST FOODS

Product	Cholesterol (mg)
Arby's	
Chicken Salad Sandwich	30
Chicken Breast	57
Burger King	
Cheeseburger	48
Bacon Double Cheeseburger	104
Hardee's	
Biscuit, Sausage	29
Biscuit, Sausage, and Egg	293
Kentucky Fried Chicken	
Breast	93
Nuggets	12 each
McDonald's	
Cheeseburger	41
Quarter Pounder with Cheese	107

As you can see, there can be a vast difference within the same restaurants and even between similar foods Here is a longer list of chain restaurants and their lowest cholesterol fare:

Table 12.   LOW-CHOLESTEROL CHOICES

Product	Cholesterol (mg)
Arby's	
Chicken Salad	12
Chicken Salad Sandwich	30
French Fries	6
Roast Beef Sandwich	45
Burger King	
Apple Pie	4
Cheeseburger	48
Cherry Pie	6
Chicken Tenders	47
Fish Filet	43
Hamburger	37
French Fries	14
Hardee's	
Apple Turnover	5
Biscuit, Gravy	21
Biscuit, Sausage	29
Biscuit, Ham	17
Cheeseburger	28
French Fries	4
Hamburger	22
Hash Rounds	10
Jack in the Box	
Club Pita	43
French Fries	8
Taco, regular	21
Taco, super	37
Kentucky Fried Chicken	
Nuggets	12
Baked Beans	1
Buttermilk Biscuit	1
Coleslaw	4
Corn on the Cob	1
Mashed Potatoes	1
Long John Silver	
Fried Fish	31

Product	Cholesterol (mg)
Fried Shrimp	17
Coleslaw	12
Hushpuppies	1
4 pieces Chicken Plank	25
6 pieces Chicken Nugget	25
Scallop Dinner	37
McDonald's	
Biscuit with Spread	9
Biscuit with Sausage	48
Cheeseburger	41
English Muffin w/butter	15
Filet of Fish	45
French Fries	9
Hamburger	29
McDonaldland Cookie	10

Source: USDA sources.

LE CHIC CHOLESTEROL

When you go to better restaurants, with more diverse menus, a few well-chosen questions can help you decide what to order or even whether to dine there at all. Ask the maitre d' these three questions —or, better yet, call a day ahead to ask.

• *Is the food in your restaurant made to order, or is it the pre-made, heat 'em, and feed 'em variety?*: If food is made to order it can be prepared without certain ingredients if the chef allows it. But if foods are the prepackaged variety, there is little chance to alter their content before they hit the serving plate.

• *If your restaurant's food is prepared by a chef, is he or she willing to cook it to request?*: Instead of frying foods, is the chef willing to bake, boil, steam, or poach what he or she is cooking? Will he or she use vegetable or olive oil in place of butter in preparation? Will he or she leave salt out of a meal on request? How about MSG, which is very high in sodium? What about gravies and sauces, which are almost always high in fat?

• *Can meat portions be limited to 4 to 6 ounces?* If you like to clean your plate, it's better not to have so much to clean. Rather than a 12-ounce New York cut, ask the restaurant if it will serve half that amount. Can all visible fat be trimmed from meat and poultry before it is broiled or baked? Between the trimming and the cooking fire, much of the fat can be removed from the meat.

A final tip: order fruit instead of pastry or other fattening desserts.

You may be surprised to find many restaurants happy to accommodate your requests. Some chefs consider low-fat, low-cholesterol cooking an art in itself.

Minding the Menu

But what do you do on those occasions when you find yourself eating in an unaccommodating restaurant? You can learn to "read" a menu. Look for these important low-fat words: steamed, poached, prepared in its own juices, garden fresh, broiled, fresh, clear (as in clear broth), broasted, roasted, dry broiled, raw (as in "raw vegetables"), grilled, margarine, vegetable oil, olive oil.

Be sure to avoid foods with these words: stewed, basted, deep-fried, au gratin, cheese sauce, escalloped, creamed, cream sauce, creamy (as in creamy dressing), in its own gravy, hollandaise, marinated in oil, prime, hash, pot pie, buttery, butter sauce, sautéed, fried, crispy, braised, pan-fried, casserole, pickled, in broth, cocktail sauce, and smoked.

Ethnic Explorations

I have a friend, whom I'll call Jay, who loves to eat in restaurants. He's also on the Reversal Diet. I asked him about passing along his tips on eating out. Jay says he loves all kinds of cuisines, and he has developed an approach to ethnic restaurants. His rule of thumb for all of them is "keep it simple," which usually means to avoid sauces, butter, cheeses, and "hidden" fats. But being the consumate planner, he has specific suggestions.

FRENCH

Although French food is wonderful, Jay knows it is one of the great offenders in the fat and cholesterol department. By doing his home-work through the American Heart Association and nutritional anal-ysis charts like the one included in Chapter 3, Jay assembled a list of "preferred" French cuisine.

Choose "nouvelle" sauces, if sauce you must: Sauces are the heart of French cuisine, and they present difficulties to the reversal dieter. Typical sauces such as hollandaise, béarnaise, and béchamel include egg yolks, butter, milk, and a considerable amount of salt. These ingredients add up to a whopping cholesterol count. Two tablespoons of hollandaise, for instance, contain 128 milligrams of cholesterol. The same amount of béarnaise sauce has 106 milligrams.

If for some reason sauces can't be put on the side (and there is really no reason a restaurant shouldn't be able to accommodate that re-quest), then the nouvelle sauces should be the order of the day. They are lighter and sometimes contain no cholesterol or milk products. Jay is always sure to ask what they contain before he orders.

Ask for French country cooking: The simplest form of French cook-ing is country style. The food is often cooked in its own juices only, with wine and spices being added for flavor. If there is sauce, put it on the side, s'il vous plaît.

Try cheese-less onion soup: Jay is in the habit of ordering his French onion soup without cheese. There isn't much he can do about the high sodium content of the soup (except not eat it), but he figures that by leaving the cheese off, at least he gets rid of the fat.

GREEK

Greek food can be a blessing and a curse for the reversal dieter. The Greeks have a diet filled with simple foods and the monounsaturated oil of the olive, which is thought to protect against heart disease. That is why people in the countries around the Mediterranean have a lower rate of heart disease than those in many other countries, most notably the United States. However, feta cheese and anchovies are danger areas. Both are very high in sodium, and the feta is also high in fat. The phyllo dough used in many entrées and desserts is also high in fat. And caviar, frequently used in appetizers, is high in cholesterol.

Preferred Greek dishes: Now when Jay eats Greek, he orders veg-etable dishes and shish kabob (light on the lamb). Pita breads are great because they are low in fat, and of course dishes prepared with olive oil are fine as long as they aren't too oily.

INDIAN

With the exception of fried breads, Jay found a lot of safety in Indian cuisine. On the whole it is low in saturated fat, cholesterol, and calories if certain choices are avoided.

For instance, some of the dishes use a yogurt-based sauce, which is fine if the yogurt is low-fat. However, some breads and many of the vegetables are fried. Jay knows he has to avoid the fried breads because they soak up the fatty oil in the frying process. But the fried vegetables are fine if only a small amount of vegetable oil is used.

Preferred Indian fare: With those exceptions, the Indian menu is fine. Breads like the unleavened wheat bread called pulkas are without cholesterol and saturated fat and are excellent alone, without butter or margarine.

Other excellent choices are the fish dishes and tandoori chicken, which are roasted in a clay pot after being marinated in spices. Shish kebab, a marinated lamb cooked over hot coals, is a great meal if the lamb is lean and less of it is used.

ITALIAN

The possibilities of Italian cuisine make those restaurants a good choice for Jay, too. All he has to do is make sure the foods he orders aren't full of cheeses or meats and the pasta isn't tossed with cream sauces or butter.

Italian foods of choice: Jay avoids sauces with meat, because he knows such fare will put him way over his cholesterol and saturated-fat numbers. But he knows from the nutrition tables that virtually any sauce without meat is acceptable. He is amazed at how many of those there are. There are marinara and marsala (made with wine), or linguine with clam sauce. He realizes that he can even have pasta primavera and fresh vegetables if he can convince the kitchen to go light on the oil.

Jay found another plus in an Italian restaurant—dessert. Not only can he usually have fresh fruit, but Jay also discovered Italian ices. No cholesterol, no fat, but very tasty.

ORIENTAL

Of all the kinds of ethnic restaurants, Jay found the Japanese to be the safest for the reversal dieter. All those raw-fish delights such as sashimi and sushi contain Omega-3 oils that are actually good for his heart.

Although he avoids anything deep-fried such as tempura and the soups that are high in sodium, Jay can eat anything else freely.

Jay found Japanese food to be the reversal dieter's dream.

The same was true of Chinese food, with some exceptions. Egg foo yung, for instance, is not a reversal food because its eggs, of course, contain cholesterol. Lobster sauce is on the black list because it, too, contains copious amounts of cholesterol. Beef, pork, and especially those fatty duck dishes are passed by in favor of chicken and vegetable choices. And, of course, deep-fried foods in a Chinese restaurant are to be as carefully avoided as they are in a fast-food restaurant.

Even though those items are out of the question, Jay is left with many choices. When he orders, he is careful to ask that no MSG be used so the sodium level of the food can be kept to a minimum. The same is true of the soy sauce, which he has learned to live without.

MEXICAN

If food from the Orient is the reversal dieter's dream, then food from Mexico is his nightmare. Refried beans and corn tortillas sound like perfect reversal food, but when Jay found out that most foods in Mexican restaurants contain lard, he knew he had eaten his last bean burrito. Since cheese, sauces, and meats are to be avoided, Jay felt there might be very little for him to eat at a Mexican restaurant.

South of the border reversal food: But Jay made some discoveries about Mexican food that preserve the experience for him. Corn tortillas that are baked (not fried) usually contain no lard. Don't be afraid to ask how they are prepared. Salads, especially those with a Mexican flair such as tomato, onion, and avocado, can be enjoyed with fresh lemon squeezed on top.

Seviche, a fish marinated in lime juice, makes a fine appetizer. And if hunger still persists, Jay can always order a chicken or shrimp tostada on an unfried corn tortilla. With salsa poured on top, the only difference between this modified order and the regular one is the crunch of deep-fried corn.

The Plan Works

If you're someone who does business at lunch or dinner or breakfast—
or at all three!—by planning ahead, you can lose weight, reduce your
cholesterol level, bring your blood pressure well within a safe range,
and still impress your clients and associates. As I hope I've shown,
you can eat well and still eat heart-healthy foods in almost any restaurant.

EXERCISE

Perhaps nothing has a greater effect upon the reversal of heart disease than regular exercise. And I don't mean the strenuous regimen necessary to train marathon runners or long-distance swimmers. Although these athletes are a living testament to the heart's strength, the amount of exercise they do is far more than you need to do to achieve reversal.

Small amounts of regular exercise have a great effect upon the cardiovascular system. Exercise lowers serum-cholesterol levels. It increases the amount of HDL cholesterol, the kind that cleans the bad LDL cholesterol out of the arteries. It helps lower blood pressure. It reduces total body fat. It improves your mental state.

But perhaps most important is the *functional reversal* that results from exercise. Exercise makes the heart beat stronger. That is important. Even though a heart may be impaired by coronary artery disease, it can often compensate for these weaknesses by the strength that exercise gives it. You might compare this to an eight-fingered piano player who plays as well as his ten-fingered counterparts. He can't grow back the two lost fingers and *anatomically* reverse his situation, but he can *functionally* improve by training the fingers that he has.

It's the same with the heart. The anatomically impaired heart can usually be trained with exercise to improve functionally. This is only true to a point, of course, and this is one reason a doctor should be consulted before starting any regular exercise program. However keep in mind that it is the doctors who are sometimes the problem when it comes to physical activity. In fact, worsening atherosclerosis is often due to the Five D's: Disease, Disuse, Drugs, and Damned Doctors. I say "Damned Doctors" because they restrict people. If a doctor says you shouldn't be active, don't be afraid to get a second opinion. What Hippocrates said about the power of exercise is usually true: *All parts of the body which have a function, if used in moderation and exercised in labors in which each is accustomed, become thereby healthy, well-developed, and age more slowly, but if unused and left idle they become liable to disease, defective in growth, and age quickly.* In other words, be active and don't spend a lot of time in bed—unless you are being active there, too.

The ability of exercise to reverse heart disease functionally became clear to me in 1950, when I began developing the concept of exercise therapy for coronary heart disease. In the years leading up to that development, people who'd had heart attacks were considered disabled. Corporations often "retired" them early on the advice of the corporate doctors. These heart-attack victims—many of them young men—were thought to be too close to death's door to do a day's work. As a result they became inactive, bored, and depressed. They believed what the doctors were saying, that they were at the end of their lives with an incurable disease. No one thought of heart disease as being a reversible condition.

The truth may not have been discovered so soon had World War II not created a need for manpower. With so many men serving overseas, the government was desperate for workers. To see if heart-attack victims could be put back to work, Dr. Leonard Goldwater of New York's Bellevue Hospital was asked to examine a sizable number of patients with coronary heart disease. To everyone's surprise, he found that many of the patients he examined were functionally well enough to return to work. They were simply being led to believe that they were disabled by their doctors.

In 1950, the American Heart Association decided to carry the study of heart patients further. They asked me to establish the Work Classification Clinic, a program designed simply to find out how to get a person with heart disease back to work.

I hired vocational counselors and a psychiatric social worker to help deal with the emotional problems sometimes created by heart disease, those feelings of anger and despair some patients have about a body that has "failed" them. I also recruited an exercise physiologist to do what no one had done before—to see how much energy was actually being expended by the heart when a person was working.

We tested and followed 2,973 people with heart disease. We discovered many things about the way heart patients live and work. Among them was this: *On the whole, people don't work hard enough to tax their hearts.* We may feel tired at the end of the day. But few of us increase our heart rates to a level that could be considered exercise.

For instance, some of the heart patients we studied could not walk on a treadmill for a minute and a half, yet they were holding down jobs in heavy industry, doing as much work as healthier men. The reason for this apparent contradiction: the treadmills were forcing them to use their hearts to full capacity. Work wasn't. In fact, I found that it takes more energy to clean house than it does to work in most factories!

Up until that point the medical world thought of work as a cause of heart attacks, something that would kill a heart patient if continued. We found that most workers used only about one-fourth of their cardiovascular capacity. We also found that it was *lack* of work that was killing heart patients.

This was a new way of looking at heart disease, and it inspired me to examine the benefits of exercise on the wounded heart. I helped organize the National Exercise and Heart Disease Project to see if exercise could help heart patients recover. This revolutionary study monitored 651 patients across the nation as they helped us explore new ground, something we called *cardiac rehabilitation.*

For two years these patients exercised three times a week, an hour each time. Everything they did during these sessions was monitored with electrodes to make certain that they exercised at 85 percent of their maximum heart rate. At the end of the study, we had at least functionally reversed the heart disease of almost every subject by making their heart muscle stronger and able to perform better. We had also uncovered many of the benefits of exercise that make it a sort of "magic pill" in the reversal of heart disease:

• **Regular exercise reduces serum cholesterol:** We found that regular exercise lowers serum cholesterol. In our patients, cholesterol levels dropped enough to make a significant difference in mortality and the rate of recurring heart attack.

Our findings have been confirmed by many researchers and has been shown to happen even without dietary intervention.

Why does exercise reduce total cholesterol? M. René Malinow found the answer when he "tagged" cholesterol with small amounts of radioactivity and fed it to rats that were then exercised on treadmills. Tests revealed radioactivity in the carbon dioxide that they exhaled. This meant simply that the cholesterol was being burned as fuel, which is one reason exercisers have less of it.

• **Exercise creates HDL, or "good" cholesterol:** In our study group, HDL increased. Other studies have replicated these results. One published in the *Journal of the American Medical Association* showed that

HDL increased as much as 10 percent in ten marathon runners after they ran a race. Another study conducted by Dr. Linn Goldberg at the Oregon Health Sciences University showed that even weight lifting, a nonaerobic exercise, reduces the amount of LDL cholesterol in the bloodstream. Even nonaerobic exercise lowers LDL.

Why does exercise have these positive effects upon HDL cholesterol and triglyceride levels in the blood? Burning fat as fuel is one way it is lowered in the bloodstream. For another it "uses up" extra fat in the body as a ready fuel.

• *Exercise reduces body fat:* Almost all of the people in our study lost weight. Granted they were following the reversal diet program, which causes weight loss in itself. But the regular exercise kept the muscle in use and prevented it from being lost along with the fat. Overall, this improved their heart function even more, since a muscular body is "living weight" that helps the heart do its job of pumping blood. Fat, on the other hand, is "dead" weight. The more extra weight you carry around, the greater the load on your heart and circulatory system.

Many other studies (perhaps hundreds) have shown that exercise reduces body fat. Perhaps the most amazing thing in all of this is that active people eat more than those who are inactive—another benefit of exercise.

• *Exercise improves oxygen uptake in muscle:* In addition to the exercised body being leaner, the trained muscle is also better at extracting oxygen from the bloodstream. This is caused by a rise in *oxidative enzymes* in the skeletal muscle. These enzymes lower heart rate because they allow muscles to extract oxygen more efficiently from the bloodstream.

I liken this to a supply boat that has a limited amount of time to unload food at a town before it has to go down river to the next town. The town with the stronger villagers will be able to remove the most food from the boat, just as the muscles with the most oxidative enzymes will be able to remove the most oxygen from the blood as it passes by on its journey back to the heart.

• *Exercise lowers the amount of adrenaline in the bloodstream:* Unfit people have higher heart rates, in part because they have more adrenaline in their bloodstream than exercisers. This is because unfit people release more adrenaline to perform a given task than do fit people.

If you exercise, not only do you have less adrenaline in your blood-stream, but what you do have is put to better use. Rather than having it float around causing increased heart rate, anxiety, and worst of all, arterial damage, the well-exercised heart uses adrenaline to improve its stroke volume.

I equate high levels of adrenaline to sitting at a stop light and racing your engine while waiting for the light to change. You are expending a lot of fuel but not getting much mileage.

A high level of adrenaline does many things that contribute to the buildup of atherosclerosis. It damages the delicate intimal cells that line your blood vessels and gives artery disease a place to start. It makes the blood cells stick together and then clot on a rough or damaged spot on the artery. It even frees fatty acids, which cloud the bloodstream with fat and make it more difficult for oxygen to get to the heart.

When levels of adrenaline are reduced through exercise, much of the damage caused by free-floating adrenaline is reversed.

• *Exercise lowers blood pressure:* We found that virtually all of our patients lowered their blood pressure to the reversal range.

This didn't surprise anyone in the medical community. As early as the 1930s it was known that athletes had lower blood pressure than people who were sedentary.

More recently, Dr. Ralph Paffenbarger of Stanford University showed that strenuous leisure-time exercise lowers blood pressure. He examined the life-style habits of 17,000 Harvard alumni and found that the chances of having hypertension were 20 to 40 percent lower in active individuals.

These studies also showed that exercise makes your heart beat more slowly when it is at rest. This slower resting pulse rate is merely a reflection of a stronger heart that is able to pump blood more efficiently. Both slower heart rate and lower blood pressure have been shown independently to slow and reverse atherosclerosis in experimental animals.

Exercise may also help lower blood pressure by increasing the pliability of the arteries, making them less rigid. It certainly increases the diameter of the main coronary arteries. Although increasing the size of these coronary arteries doesn't necessarily lower blood pressure, it does allow a greater amount of blood to flow to the heart, even through arteries that may be partially blocked with plaque.

• *Exercise creates collateral circulation:* Studies show that vigorous exercise stimulates the growth of capillaries from the main coronary arteries to feed more blood to the heart. This capillary growth, known as *collateral circulation,* develops when the heart muscle has a consistent need for more oxygen than it normally gets through coronary artery blood flow. This increased demand causes the cells to release enzymes that stimulate the growth of capillaries. Sometimes these capillaries are already there but are empty because they aren't needed.

Increased collateral circulation can occur when arteries are slowly choked by atherosclerosis. In essence, these new capillaries function as a natural bypass, a way for blood to get around the blockage and feed the heart muscle that would otherwise die for lack of oxygen. Of course if the blockage occurs very quickly, collaterals don't have time to form or open and a heart attack occurs.

The demands of exercise also create collateral circulation *around* the heart. Dr. Richard Eckstein dramatically demonstrated this when he narrowed the left-circumflex coronary artery in several dogs and exercise-trained half the group. He then compared the collateral flow in the exercised group to that of the nonexercised and found the additional flow in the exercisers to be enormous. He then carried the research further. In some of the animals from each group he completely closed the circumflex artery. Few of the exercised animals died, and if they lost heart muscle they lost much less than the nonexercised control animals did.

In humans I have seen collaterals as large as a millimeter in diameter, reaching across the heart from a "clear" artery to feed an area blocked and not getting normal blood flow.

How quickly can blood begin flowing through these collateral "channels" that are ready to be used when increased demand calls for it? Doctors here at Case Western showed that by reducing blood flow approximately 50 percent through the anterior descending artery of dogs and waiting only one hour, the artery could then be closed the rest of the way and only 10 out of 100 dogs would die of a heart attack! The remaining 90 had enough collateral blood flow to keep their hearts alive!

Vigorous exercise opens these collaterals by creating a greater oxygen demand in the heart. This bonus blood flow is part of the reason a well-exercised heart beats slower and more efficiently.

Table 13 from *Cardiovascular Review & Reports* examines the out-
come of eleven major studies on exercise and heart disease. As you
can see, the more active the study subjects, the lower their risk of
coronary heart disease.

Table 13.   PHYSICAL ACTIVITY AND CORONARY DISEASE

Study Group	Number of Subjects	Length of Study Period (years)	Method of Quantification of Physical Activity	Outcome
Retrospective Studies				
London busmen, 1953	31,000	2	Job title	Sedentary workers had double the incidence of new angina, MI, and death but also more high BP, cholesterol, and obesity
Israeli kibbutzim, 1960	8,500	10	Job description	Sedentary workers had three times the incidence of MI in a population with nearly uniform diet and environment
American railroad workers, 1962	192,000	2	Job title	Men in sedentary jobs had twice the age-adjusted coronary death rate as men in active jobs
American postal employees, 1963	2,240	34	Job title	Sedentary postal clerks had 1.4–1.9 times the CHD mortality risk of active letter carriers
Health Insurance Plan, New York, 1966	301 first MI	1.5	Interview	Three times higher MI case fatality rate in least vs most active subjects
London busmen, 1966	667	5	Job title	Sedentary busdrivers had 1.8 times the incidence of CHD of active conductors

Study Group	Number of Subjects	Length of Study Period (years)	Method of Quantification of Physical Activity	Outcome
Framingham, 1967	5,127	—	Interviews and assessment of weight gain, vital capacity, and resting heart rate	Most sedentary had five times the CHD mortality of most active
Chicago gas company workers, 1970	1,241	7	Job description	Blue collar (active) workers had lower CHD mortality, but other risk factors could account for difference
British civil servants, 1973	16,882	5	Questionnaire, weekend activities diary	Men recording vigorous exercise had 50% subsequent incidence of those who did not record vigorous exercise
San Francisco longshoremen, 1975	6,351	22	Job assignments with caloric work output computations	Low activity workers had 1.8 times the CHD mortality, especially sudden death, of high activity workers
Harvard alumni, 1978	16,936	6–10	Questionnaire, with caloric output computed (physical activity index)	Men with physical activity index <2,000 kcal/wk had 64% greater risk of first MI than classmates with higher index— independent of most other risk factors

CHD = coronary heart disease; MI = myocardial infarction; BP = blood pressure; NS = nonsignificant.
Source: R. Fuchs, M.D., "Prevention of Coronary Atherosclerosis," part I. *Cardiovascular Review & Reports*, May 1983, p. 793.

Getting Results

The goal of the National Exercise and Heart Disease Project was to study the effects of exercise and other life-style changes on heart disease. The results were remarkable, more conclusive than any of the doctors or patients involved really expected. We had changed the risk factors for cardiovascular disease so greatly that we reversed the heart disease of many of these patients. Exercise had reduced the chance of mortality in these heart-attack victims by 37 percent.

EXERCISE RECOMMENDATION:
TO GET FIT, RELY ON F.I.T.

Many of you might cringe at the thought of exercise because you think of it as "boring," "work," or "a waste of time." The fact is that exercise can be all or none of those. What is important can be summed up in one simple rule: keep it fun.

Fun exercise is the type you do on a regular basis without it seeming like "boring" "work" that is "a waste of time." I subscribe to the words of the Earl of Derby, who almost a century ago said: "Those who think they have not time for bodily exercise will sooner or later have to find time for illness."

Although exercise done at a greater intensity usually has a more positive effect upon the heart, most of the benefits of exercise can be attained through any of its forms, including walking upstairs instead of taking an elevator or parking at the far end of the parking lot when you go to the shopping center.

The value of this kind of background exercise has been demonstrated in several excellent studies. In Dr. Paffenbarger's study of the physical activity of 17,000 Harvard alumni, he found that longevity increased with activity, with death rates declining steadily as energy expended on such things as walking and stair climbing increased. He found that people who play vigorous sports had the lowest death rates, but right behind them were people who were active but didn't necessarily work up a sweat.

Exactly what is exercise worth in terms of added life? Paffenbarger found that for every hour spent working out, a person adds approximately an hour to his life. And that is a tangible benefit beyond the improved psychological well-being that exercise brings and the added energy it contributes to daily living.

Picking up those extra hours of life can be easy, relatively painless, and, of course, fun. Ride a bicycle or walk to your commuting station. Sell your riding lawn mower. Get rid of the upstairs telephone. Fire your gardener. Jog in place during the evening news. Get rid of your chainsaw and chop firewood by hand. These are just some of the more obvious ways of increasing activity in your daily life.

But as beneficial as background exercise is, I still don't think it can take the place of a regular exercise program. To gain all of the reversal benefits of exercise and maintain them, a regular workout routine needs to become a part of your life. But once again, it has to be fun.

I can't tell you what kind of exercise to do. You have to decide which exercise is fun and which isn't. Even gardening is exercise and if done on a regular basis it can be considered part of your regular exercise routine.

The point of this is to do some type of exercise, and do it according to the principles of F.I.T., or Frequency, Intensity, and Time. Whatever exercise you choose, following the F.I.T. principles will ensure that you are getting the exercise you need to help put your vital numbers into the reversal range.

It is also a good idea to learn to read the signs your body gives you when it is being overexercised. If you experience muscle soreness that doesn't go away quickly, decrease the amount of exercise you are doing until the soreness disappears. Other signs of overexercising are fitful sleep, frequent urination, an elevated resting pulse rate, and a rapid weight loss. All of these are indications that your metabolism has speeded up and your body is trying to recover from too much working out. Reduce your level of exercise if these signs appear.

The heart has a language of its own when it comes to overwork. If you feel dizzy or have chest pains while exercising, stop immediately and see your doctor. The same goes for pains in the jaw and in the arms. These areas are often the first to feel pain if the heart isn't pumping properly because they are not getting sufficient blood. If these areas ache, stop exercising and see your doctor, too.

Before beginning a regular exercise program I recommend seeing a doctor for an exercise stress test. Not only will it give you peace of mind about the health of your cardiovascular system, but it will also provide a baseline test of fitness against which you can show improvement.

With all that in mind, here are the F.I.T. principles:

• **Frequency:** Exercise should be done at least three times per week, according to the American College of Sportsmedicine. Doing a specific activity three times per week gives you a chance to have a day off in between to recover from muscle soreness. When you are ready to increase frequency there is no harm in going up to four, five, or even seven days of exercise. Three days a week is merely a minimum standard established by the ACSM.

• **Intensity:** The ACSM recommends that exercise be done at 60 to 90 percent of maximum heart rate. For people with suspected or diagnosed heart disease, I prefer that 60 to 85 percent of the highest heart rate obtained during a medically supervised exercise test be used. Although Paffenbarger's study shows that activity of any kind—regardless of intensity—increases longevity, I think there are certain reversal factors to be gained through intensity. For one, the greater the intensity, the greater the strengthening of the heart. Also, collateral circulation is more likely to build when there is greater demand for oxygen in the heart muscle.

Intensity is reflected in the heart rate—the greater the heart rate, the greater the intensity.

To find your "target heart-rate zone," subtract your age from 220 if you are normal. That number is your maximum heart rate, as measured in beats per minute. Then multiply that number by .60 to .90 to find the heart rate and intensity you are trying to sustain.

For example, if you are 40 years old, subtract your age from 220 to get your maximum heart rate—180. Then multiply this figure by .60 and .90 to find your target range—a pulse rate of 108 to 162 beats per minute.

Table 14 lists target heart rates for normal subjects of various ages:

Table 14. TARGET HEART RATES

Age	Target Range (60% to 90%)	Age	Target Range (60% to 90%)
25	117–175	55	99–148
30	114–171	60	96–144
35	111–166	65	93–139
40	108–162	70	90–135
45	105–157	75	87–130
50	102–153	80	84–126

To measure your heart rate during a workout, stop exercising for a moment and place two fingers on your neck right below your ear, or on your wrist. Your heartbeat is stronger and much easier to find during exercise. Count the number of beats in ten seconds and multiply that number by six to get the count for one minute. That will provide your heart rate for one minute.

After doing this a number of times, you will begin to sense when you are in the target zone and will not need to take your pulse.

• *Time:* The ACSM recommends at least 20 to 30 minutes of exercise per session. But again, this is the minimum amount suggested to benefit your heart. People exercise many times this long and receive many times the benefit. But for minimum heart fitness, at least twenty minutes per session is required.

GETTING WITH IT, STAYING WITH IT

As the F.I.T. principles show, exercise doesn't have to be painful or boring for you to reap its reversal benefits. That is good news for many people who want to start but are afraid to do so for a variety of reasons.

Keep in mind, though, that it is important to have a plan of attack before beginning an exercise program. Research shows that it is much easier to drop out of a program than it is to start and stay with one. When I recommend regular exercise to a patient, I offer these specific guidelines to help him or her to get started and stay with it:

• *Make your exercise goals realistic:* Many people begin an exercise program with great expectations. They try to swim thirty laps in an Olympic-sized pool, or to duplicate the New York City Marathon after seeing it on TV. Such high hopes are likely to bring your exercise program to an abrupt halt. Fitness specialists recommend concentrating on time spent exercising rather than on intensity. As long as you are breathing more heavily, that's fine, since that probably means that your heart rate is somewhere within the target range.

• *Find the right time:* Early-morning workouts give some people a lift in energy and mood that lasts all day. Others prefer to exercise after work to release the day's tensions. Psychotherapists recommend exercising regularly at the time of the day when you're most anxious, to defuse your anxiety. The key: Get your exercise at the time that suits you best. The Toronto Life Assurance Study showed that 46 percent of 1,800 subjects said they had quit exercising because they thought they didn't have time.

• *Vary your exercise routine:* This is especially important if you're among those who find exercise boring. And don't feel guilty if you are. Close to 90 percent of people polled at the 1980 Ironman Triathlon began training for swimming, bicycling, and running because they were bored with just one sport. If people at that high level of fitness are bored, it is safe to project that people less devoted to exercise have even more boredom in their ranks and need variety for stimulation.

• *Plot your progress:* Keep track of your achievements with a diary, like the one in this book. And reward yourself. Reward is especially important in the early stages of an exercise program, before exercise becomes a pleasure in itself. Even some champion athletes reward themselves with meals or other treats for good training sessions. But simple things like words of encouragement can help a novice over the hump and into a world of joyful exercise.

• *Keep it fun:* Exercisers who were encouraged to think distracting or pleasant thoughts ("go slow and smell the flowers") were more likely to stick with an exercise program than subjects trained to focus on "body sensations" (i.e., pain) and challenging goals, found clinical psychologist John Martin of San Diego State University. Boredom, by contrast, drove 20 percent of the exercise dropouts in the Toronto Life Assurance Study to give up their workouts.

Finally, it is good to remember the words of Moses Maimonides, the tenth-century philosopher/physician whose words have had a profound effect upon medicine, even today. *The most beneficial of all types of exercise is physical gymnastics to the point that the soul becomes influenced and rejoices.* In other words, do the kind of exercise that you like. And if you don't like it, do something else. As you can see from the chart below, there is more than one way to burn a calorie.

Table 15. AVERAGE NUMBER OF CALORIES BURNED IN EXERCISE PER MINUTE				
	Weight in Pounds			
Activity	105–115	127–137	160–170	182–192
Bicycling (stationary)	11	13	15	17
Trampolining	10	11	13	15
Skiing, X-C	9	10	12	13
Running	9	10	12	13
Jogging	8	9	11	12

Activity	Weight in Pounds			
	105–115	127–137	160–170	182–192
Snow shoveling	7	9	11	12
Volleyball	8	9	11	12
Handball	8	9	11	12
Basketball	7	8	10	11
Stair climbing	6	7	8	9
Aerobic dance	6	7	8	9
Tennis, doubles	6	6	8	8
Dancing, square	6	6	8	8
Bicycling, slow	6	6	7	7
Sawing wood	5	6	7	8
Gardening	5	6	7	8
Calisthenics	4	5	7	8
Skating	5	5	6	7
Badminton	5	5	6	7
Swimming	4	5	5	6
Sexual intercourse	4	5	5	6
Rowing	4	5	5	6
Hiking	4	5	5	6
Walking	4	5	5	6
Baseball	4	4	5	5
Lawn mowing, power	4	4	5	5
Golf	3	4	4	5
Dancing, rock	3	4	4	5

TAMERS
OF ANGRY
BLOOD

*Vitamins,
Minerals—
and Aspirin*

8

T here is no question that the proper balance of vitamins and minerals are necessary for a healthy heart. But on the whole, I don't support the belief of some nutritionists who think that mega-doses of micronutrients are a cure for what ails us. But I do subscribe to the beliefs of my former colleague, Dr. Irvine Page, who said: "I take one multi-vitamin pill in the morning largely because it . . . acts as an old-fashioned exorcist."

Actually, that multivitamin might represent more than "an old-fashioned exorcist." It is clear from the data that a diet rich in vitamins and minerals is beneficial to a healthy heart and may even help the process of reversal. Let's take a look at the vitamins first:

VITAMIN E: THE "GREAT HOPE" REEMERGES

Through the years, vitamin E (alpha tocopherol acetate) has been the "great hope" of the vitamin world. This fat-soluble vitamin has been touted as being everything from the savior of a fading sex life to a performance enhancer for athletes, only to fail on these accounts when undergoing stringent medical tests.

As Milton Scott wrote of vitamin E in *The Handbook of Lipid Research:* "One group claims that vitamin E is the cure for almost every disease known to man; the other group takes the stand that vitamin E has not been proved scientifically to have any of the effects being claimed for it. The true value of vitamin E lies between the two extremes."

Perhaps the best research on vitamin E relates to its effects upon peripheral vascular disease, the blockages that build up in a person's arms and legs. Patients in one study who were given large daily doses of vitamin E for twenty to twenty-five months had an almost 40 percent increase in blood flow to the lower legs, while the untreated control group had a 20 percent decrease.

To my knowledge, the people with the most vitamin E experience in a clinical setting are the Shute doctors in Windsor, Canada. They have treated more than 30,000 heart-disease patients with megadoses of the vitamin. They claim that their treatment—which amounts to taking 1,500 to 3,000 units of vitamin E per day—results in greatly improved blood circulation. But since they do not perform randomized controlled studies of blood flow to the heart muscle, the value of what the Shutes do cannot be weighed by the medical community.

In my own practice, however, I have had patients whose leg cramps have been greatly relieved by doses of vitamin E. But this is just my personal observation; I have never conducted a study on the reversal properties of vitamin E nor do I know of anyone who has.

RECOMMENDATION: 10 MG PER DAY. BUT . . .

I recommend a vitamin E intake of 10 mg per day, an amount easily provided by the foods in the reversal diet. Despite some interesting research and observations regarding this vitamin, I don't think benefits of larger doses than these have been sufficiently proved—yet. The future may certainly prove that this is too small a dose to fight all the oxidants we are exposed to today. In addition to the foods in our deep-fried society, the pollution of modern living contributes greatly to the number of oxidants or "free radicals" our bodies have to contend with. The antioxidant properties of vitamins like E might bind with these free radical molecules, keeping them from damaging cells. Research in the next few years might bring vitamin E to the fore in the contribution of micronutrients to the fight against heart disease. But right now, without sufficient data to back supplementation, I will stick with the RDA provided by the fine research of the federal government.

But for people who want to take supplements and achieve at least a placebo effect (if not more) the Food and Nutrition Board of the National Research Council has some advice. In 1980 they produced research showing that a daily vitamin E dose of 150 to 350 mg did not adversely affect most adults. And since toxic effects are minimal, you can be the judge as to whether or not to supplement the reversal diet with vitamin E.

But before you buy those capsules, you might want to read the food tables below to get an idea of how many milligrams are found in some reversal foods:

Table 16. VITAMIN E IN REVERSAL FOODS			
Food	Vitamin E (mg)	Food	Vitamin E (mg)
Corn oil (1 tbsp)	3.00	Almonds, dried (1 oz)	6.75
Cottonseed oil (1 tbsp)	4.80	Asparagus (4 spears)	1.15
Sunflower oil (1 tbsp)	6.10	Pasta, cooked (1 cup)	1.03
Wheat germ oil (1 tbsp)	20.30	Spinach, boiled (½ cup)	2.70
Mazola margarine, diet (1 tbsp)	8.00		

VITAMIN C, THE SOUR DO-ALL

Like vitamin E, vitamin C has long been touted as the "do all" supplement. Vitamin C, or "ascorbic acid," prevents and cures scurvy, a painful and sometimes fatal disease in which joints swell and wounds don't heal. It also aids in the absorption of iron and helps the body recover from infections. For a while there was hope that vitamin C could stop or reverse atherosclerosis. But studies have shown these hopes to be false.

Although lack of vitamin C might raise cholesterol levels, there is no good indication that larger than normal doses can reduce serum cholesterol.

Some of the misunderstanding about vitamin C and cholesterol reduction might stem from the fact that fruit and vegetable consumption in this country has risen since 1968, the year that deaths from heart disease began falling. Although some researchers attributed this drop in death rate to increased levels of vitamin C in the diet, they failed to account for one factor: the consumption of more fruits and vegetables means that fewer foods containing cholesterol and saturated fats will be eaten. Also, the fiber in fruits and vegetables is a natural bile sequestrant that binds with bile acids as it passes from the body. Fruits and vegetables also speed the transit time of the bowel and thereby increase the loss of cholesterol.

The antioxidant properties of vitamin C put it in the same mysterious league with the other free-radical tamers.

Animals, such as the guinea pig, and humans who are unable to synthesize vitamin C showed a significant rise in serum cholesterol when deprived of vitamin C. Researcher E. Ginter found an increase in serum cholesterol of 44 percent after twenty weeks of vitamin C restriction. Other researchers have shown increases in the range of 75 to 100 percent. This isn't surprising since vitamin C is needed to convert cholesterol into cholic acid, one of the main components of bile.

Since vitamin C is necessary for the production of collagen, a protein found in all connecting tissues including blood vessels, it is also no surprise that vitamin C deprivation can cause the breakdown of the arterial walls.

Once again, E. Ginter showed that the arteries of vitamin C-deprived guinea pigs had damage to the intimal cells of the endothelial layer. The reason for the damage was a lack of new collagen, one of the body's building blocks.

As an antioxidant, vitamin C protects some vitamins and fatty acids from being oxidized. Since cholesterol is a form of alcohol, vitamin C may protect the arteries by preventing the oxidation of cholesterol. That is purely speculation at this point. As further research examines the connection between free radicals and heart disease, vitamin C may achieve status as a heart-healing vitamin. But until then I'll stick with the government's recommended requirement.

RECOMMENDATIONS: 60 MG DAILY. BUT OVERDOSING WOULD BE DIFFICULT

The National Research Council advises 60 milligrams a day, which is roughly equal to less than eight ounces of orange juice. Additional supplementation is recommended for smokers, regular aspirin users, those who take oral contraceptives, and people recovering from infections, surgery, or injury.

How much extra? 250 milligrams per day in the form of a chewable supplement would do no harm. And people frequently tolerate many times that amount, since reaching a toxic level of vitamin C would require great perseverance and a tremendous tolerance for acidity in the stomach. Since vitamin C is water soluble, it does not collect in body fat but is excreted in urine.

Be forewarned, however, that high levels of vitamin C have been linked to kidney stones and loss of red blood cells.

But before you reach for the bottle of ascorbic acid, take a look at some of the reversal foods below that are high in vitamin C. In addition to whatever ascorbic acid you want, these foods provide fiber (which lowers cholesterol), potassium (which improves blood pressure), and many of the vitamins and minerals you may be thinking of taking in bottle form.

Table 17.   VITAMIN C IN REVERSAL FOODS

Food	Vitamin C (mg)	Food	Vitamin C (mg)
Fruit		Raspberries (1 cup)	31
Apple (1)	12	Raspberry juice (1 cup)	41
Banana (1)	10	**Vegetables**	
Grapefruit (½)	41	Asparagus (1 cup)	49
Grapefruit juice (1 cup)	94	Broccoli (1 spear)	113
Kiwi fruit (1)	74	Cabbage (1 cup)	40
Lemon juice (1 cup)	112	Carrots (1 cup)	10
Orange (1)	70	Cauliflower (1 cup)	72
Orange juice (1 cup)	124	Red peppers (1)	141
Pineapple (1 cup)	24	Tomatoes (1)	22
Pineapple juice (1 cup)	27	Turnip greens (1 cup)	39

CAN FOLIC ACID HELP REVERSE HEART DISEASE?

The most exciting recent discovery about vitamins is the effect folic acid deficiency has on the amino acid *homocystine.* An elevated level of this amino acid, which is produced by the body, has been linked to heart disease for many years.

Genetic defects that raise homocystine levels twenty times above normal cause very early atherosclerosis, premature heart attacks, and strokes. But it was only recently that M. René Malinow and associates from the Oregon Primate Research Center began researching the link between heart disease and homocystine levels that are elevated only four or five times above normal.

His research has found that these elevations of homocystine may cause atherosclerotic heart disease *even if no other risk factors are present* —meaning persons who don't have high cholesterol levels, hypertension, or any of the other risk factors could still have coronary heart disease if they had blood levels of homocystine that were too high. So this condition, known as hyperhomocyst(e)inemia, may become an additional risk factor along with the others, and may also explain why some people get heart disease for no apparent reason.

Why is too much of this amino acid so hard on the arteries? According to a paper published by Malinow in *Circulation*, hyperhomocyst(e)inemia damages the delicate intimal cells and oxidizes (makes rancid) LDL, which allows them to enter the damaged artery lining more easily.

Malinow estimates that 20 to 25 percent of the people with heart disease have elevated homocystine levels.

Table 18. FOLIC ACID IN REVERSAL FOODS

Food	Folic Acid (mg)	Food	Folic Acid (mg)
Asparagus, fresh (½ cup)	190	Corn (½ cup)	40
Brussels sprouts (4)	130	Lentils (½ cup)	36
Chick-peas (½ cup)	125	Strawberries, fresh (1 cup)	26
Orange juice (1 cup)	110		
Wheat bran (1 oz)	80	Yogurt, low-fat (1 cup)	25
Apple (medium)	75	Carrot (1)	24
Peas, frozen (½ cup)	70	Muffin, bran	16
Pineapple juice (1 cup)	58	Milk, skim (1 cup)	15

RECOMMENDATIONS: ABOUT 400 MICROGRAMS PER DAY, BUT THAT MIGHT CHANGE

The RDA for folic acid is 400 micrograms, 0.4 milligram. This amount can easily be obtained from the reversal diet program, which favors vegetables that are fresh and grains that are unrefined. As you can see from the food chart above, high levels of folates are found in a large number of foods.

But is a daily dose of 400 micrograms of folic acid enough? In light of this new information, I don't know. Folic acid in greater amounts —even several milligrams—will not harm you, since excess amounts are simply excreted in your urine. If you are taking a multivitamin, make sure that the RDA is found in that pill. That way, the extra folic acid derived from regular food will serve to elevate your intake of this B vitamin. Or if you want, take a few milligrams of folic-acid vitamins themselves. It can't hurt, and based on the latest research, it might just help reverse coronary heart disease if you have folic acid deficiency.

THE VITAMIN/DRUG NIACIN

Vitamin B$_3$, more commonly known as niacin, plays a role in reversing coronary heart disease.

In the tiny doses received from the food we eat, this water-soluble vitamin helps the body digest fats and carbohydrates. In the much larger doses that may be prescribed by doctors, niacin opens arteries wider and reduces cholesterol levels, sometimes dramatically.

A best-selling book that offers a "cure" for cholesterol touts niacin as the wonder vitamin that lowers total cholesterol while raising the level of HDL or "good" cholesterol.

Niacin—also known as nicotinic acid and nicotinamide—certainly does all of that. Studies performed by Scott Grundy at the University of Texas Medical Center report a 22 percent reduction in cholesterol levels with the use of niacin. And the federally sponsored Coronary Drug Project, in which 1,100 patients with coronary artery blockage were given 3,000 milligrams of niacin per day, resulted in a 10 percent reduction in serum cholesterol.

But in addition to being a vitamin found in many foods, taken in large quantity niacin is also a drug with possible implications for people with heart disease, diabetes, or impaired liver function.

In fact the *Physicians' Desk Reference* warns doctors against the prescribing of niacin for people with known coronary artery disease because it can cause cardiac arrhythmias. Since many people have coronary artery disease and don't know it, I think it's important to have a complete physical and physician's approval before taking massive doses of this vitamin/drug.

RECOMMENDATION: 20 MILLIGRAMS PER DAY, WITH NIACIN SUPPLEMENTS TAKEN ONLY UNDER A DOCTOR'S SUPERVISION

Niacin has been shown to reduce serum cholesterol only in daily doses exceeding 1,000 milligrams. Doses below that have had little effect.

It is virtually impossible to get 1,000 milligrams of niacin from food —even from the foodstuffs of the reversal diet. As an example, it would take about ten peaches to provide 70 milligrams of niacin, and about 25 ounces of water-packed tuna to provide 100 milligrams. And both of those foods are high in niacin.

When niacin is gotten from food it is considered a vitamin. When it is gotten from a pill it is a drug. And the first approach I recommend with any drug is not to take it if you don't have to. In lowering cholesterol, diet therapy should be the first approach, followed by bile sequestrants. If your cholesterol still doesn't come down to a reversal level, then I recommend seeing your doctor for niacin or other therapy.

Just to satisfy any curiosity you might have, I have included a list of reversal foods that are high in niacin.

Table 19. NIACIN IN REVERSAL FOODS

Food	Niacin (mg)	Food	Niacin (mg)
Avocado (1 peeled)	5.8	Mushrooms (1 cup)	2.9
Barley (1 cup)	6.2	Peanuts (1 cup)	21.5
Breakfast cereals (1 oz)	5.0–20	Prune juice (1 cup)	2.0
Brewer's yeast (1 tbsp)	3.0	Salmon (3 oz)	5.5
Chicken (3 oz)	11.8	Sardines (3 oz)	4.6
Dates (1 cup)	3.9	Tuna, water packed (3 oz)	13.4
Halibut (3 oz)	7.7		

B_6: AN ARTERY PROTECTOR

Deficiencies of the water-soluble vitamin B_6 have been shown to induce atherosclerosis in experimental animals and speed the clotting process.

It has been reported that monkeys fed a diet low in cholesterol and fat *and* low in B_6 develop thickened arteries and lesions that look similar to those found in humans, though they are not filled with cholesterol. These results have been confirmed in several other studies as well.

When enough B_6 is in the bloodstream the clotting time of blood is prolonged. Rapidly clotting blood, as you already know, gathers on "rough spots" in the arteries and contributes greatly to atherosclerosis. When added to the feed of monkeys and dogs, B_6 has been shown to inhibit the aggregation and clotting of blood platelets.

RECOMMENDATION: 2.2 MILLIGRAMS DAILY FOR MEN, 2.0 FOR WOMEN

The few studies on B_6 and heart health confirm the importance of this vitamin. But does that mean you need to add it to your diet? If you are eating reversal foods, the answer is "no." But some studies show that the average American diet doesn't contain the 2.2 milligrams of B_6 per day that are easily consumed on the reversal diet.

For example, a study of 102 geriatric hospital patients showed that they ate less than half of the necessary B_6. And a survey of 100 adolescent girls showed that they consumed about one-third less than the RDA of this vitamin.

The reversal diet, which generally avoids processed foods, contains large quantities of B_6, as you can see in Table 20.

Some researchers feel that the RDA for B_6 is too low. And it is true that of all thirteen vitamins, B_6 is the one in which you are most likely to be deficient.

Although I don't think you need B_6 supplementation if you follow the recommendations in this book, studies have shown no side effects in daily doses of 50 to 100 milligrams. However, a lot isn't better than a little. Women who take massive doses—3,000 to 6,000 milligrams—in an attempt to relieve Premenstrual Syndrome—sometimes find themselves with numbness and shooting pains in their hands and spine. When the large doses of B_6 are stopped, the pains stop.

Table 20. VITAMIN B_6 IN REVERSAL FOODS

Food (4 oz)	B_6 (mg)	Food (4 oz)	B_6 (mg)
Brewer's yeast	4.0	Brown rice	.60
Sunflower seeds	1.36	Banana	.55
Wheat germ	1.25	Chicken	.55
Walnuts	.80	Spinach	.31
Soy flour	.66		

Minerals as Antioxidants

THE MINERAL SELENIUM

Selenium is an antioxidant that helps activate an enzyme that protects the cells of the heart, lungs, kidneys, and liver.

Maybe that is why adequate amounts of selenium have been shown to have a protective effect upon the cardiovascular system. Some small studies have shown that selenium can induce the production of prostacyclins in the arteries, a substance that relaxes them while "thinning" the blood. And in human volunteers, selenium supplementation has been shown to double the average bleeding time, which means that platelets are less prone to rapid clotting and subsequent buildup on a rough spot on an artery.

A large study examining the effects of selenium on a degenerative heart disease (cardiomyopathy) was conducted with excellent results in China. The disease, a rapid wasting of the heart muscle usually found in children and pregnant women, was so prevalent in this area of China that it was given the name of the province—Keshan.

Because the soil of the Keshan Province contains virtually no selenium, its citizens suffer from a dietary deficiency. This wasn't thought to be a problem until an outbreak of Keshan's disease led a pathologist to question the similarity between the heart muscles of one young victim and those of Australian sheep that had died mysteriously in an area of that country with low selenium content in its soil.

As a result of this pathologist's fine detective work, the Chinese government conducted a study in which they administered this mineral to over 36,000 children, while 10,000 were not given the supplement and were followed as controls.

During the four-year study, there were 21 cases and 3 deaths in the group given selenium and 107 cases and 53 deaths in the control group. Thus, selenium reduced the case rate by 95 percent and the death rate by 98 percent!

Other studies show an apparent link between adequate selenium intake and heart disease. In Finland, the risk of coronary death was found to be almost seven times greater in men with a serum selenium content lower than 34 μg/ml than in those over 45 μg/ml. Just so you'll breathe easier, the average serum level in the United States is over 100 μg/ml. The remarkable decrease in cancer of the stomach has been attributed to the widespread consumption of breakfast cereals rich in selenium.

RECOMMENDATION: 50 to 200 MICROGRAMS PER DAY

Does this apparent link between selenium and heart health mean that you should take selenium supplementation? Not on the reversal diet.

By replacing saturated fats with reversal foods like fish and whole grains, your daily dose of selenium should increase naturally to the RDA.

After all, most of the soils of America are rich in selenium. It's the processed foods that are not.

To discourage further supplementation of selenium, let me point out that high doses of this trace element are toxic. Animals that graze on selenium-laden grass become blind, lame, paralyzed, and eventually die. In humans, a toxic level would probably be around 500 micrograms per day.

Table 21 lists some examples of reversal foods that are rich in selenium.

Table 21. SELENIUM IN REVERSAL FOODS

Food	Selenium (micrograms/100 grams)	Food	Selenium (micrograms/100 grams)
Brewer's yeast	125	Garlic	25
Wheat germ	111	Oat bran	21
Wheat, whole-grain	63	Barley	18
Wheat bran	63	Mushrooms	13
Swiss chard	26		

THE MUCH-NEEDED MAGNESIUM

In other parts of this book I have referred to the role of sodium and potassium in maintaining a healthy heart. Magnesium is a mineral that plays a role in heart health, too. Deficiencies have been linked to higher rates of heartbeat irregularities, or arrhythmia; infarct, in which blood vessels constrict and reduce the flow of blood to the heart; and even atherosclerosis.

First the arrhythmia research. Many researchers have linked magnesium deficiencies to irregular heartbeat. In one such study, twenty-five patients with electrocardiogram (EKG) abnormalities were given 240 to 360 milligrams of magnesium per day. Over the two years of the study there was a pronounced reduction in the number of abnormal beats on their EKG readings. These abnormal heartbeats, called prolonged QT intervals, are often associated with sudden cardiac death.

In other studies, experimental magnesium deficiencies have led to EKG abnormalities that are related to sudden death in animals. When magnesium was returned to the diet, EKGs normalized.

Heart surgeons have effectively stopped fibrillation in patients during open-heart surgery through the use of intravenous magnesium. In the largest of these studies, heart surgeons administered IV magnesium to thirty-five patients and did not administer the mineral to a control group of the same size. The patients given the magnesium had fewer atrial fibrillations and postoperative problems than those not treated with the mineral.

Magnesium is needed by one of the enzymes of the heart to create the pumping action. When there is a deficiency, the cells have trouble pumping potassium in and sodium out, which can account for the peculiar and sometimes fatal heart rhythms.

ATHEROSCLEROSIS AND MAGNESIUM

To create atherosclerosis in experimental animals, they are fed what is called a *cardiovasopathic diet*. Typically, this diet is high in saturated fats, cholesterol, protein, sodium, phosphates, and vitamin D and low in potassium, chloride, and magnesium.

Wondering what the effects of high doses of magnesium would be on the buildup of atherosclerosis, researchers administered this diet to animals but increased the amount of magnesium to five times the usual amount. There was a slower buildup of atherosclerosis in this group than in animals fed the unsupplemented cardiovasopathic diet.

RECOMMENDATION: 350 MILLIGRAMS FOR WOMEN DAILY, 400 MILLIGRAMS FOR MEN (AT LEAST)

I accept the federal recommendation of 350 milligrams of magnesium per day for a 132-pound woman and 400 milligrams per day for a 152-pound man. Pregnant and breast-feeding women should have about 150 milligrams more per day.

Some researchers feel that the RDA for women and men should be raised to 450 milligrams and 500 milligrams, respectively, since perspiration can account for a significant loss of magnesium. Personally, I don't think magnesium deficiency is something to worry about, especially since a person on the reversal diet program will consume much more of this vital mineral than the recommended amount.

Table 22 gives the magnesium content in a few reversal foods.

Table 22. MAGNESIUM IN REVERSAL FOODS			
Food (3 oz)	Magnesium Content (mg)	Food (3 oz)	Magnesium Content (mg)
Legumes (dried)	250	Vegetables	50–100
Barley	160	Corn	35
Whole-wheat flour	140	Banana	35
Nuts	120–250	Potato	25
Brown rice	95		

One more thing about magnesium: Studies show that heart disease is generally lower in areas where drinking water is hard and contains much greater concentrations of magnesium. This finding is confirmed by some autopsy studies that show a higher concentration of magnesium in the heart muscles of people who lived in hard-water areas.

And, of Course, Aspirin

As long as we are on the subject of supplementation, we should discuss aspirin, the stuff Hippocrates brewed from the leaves of the willow tree to ease the pain of headaches and childbirth in his patients.

In 1893, the medicinal "stuff" of the willow—salicylic acid—was synthesized and modified to a more palatable form by the German chemist Felix Hoffman, and aspirin as we know it was born.

Its uses in pain relief seem to know no end. Muscle aches respond to it, fever, headaches, colds, and sinus pain; the list goes on and on for this most consumed of all drugs.

In 1988, the list grew officially longer. A number of research studies showed that aspirin could: prevent first heart attacks, help prevent a second heart attack, and greatly improve one's chances of surviving a heart attack.

Aspirin works its magic by inhibiting prostaglandin, the hormone that causes platelets to clump and clot when there is a cut or when the blood comes in contact with a rough spot such as a lesion in the artery. Since we know that clotted blood is part of the atheroma that builds up in the artery, the use of aspirin certainly contributes to the halting or the reversal of the atherosclerotic process. In the early stages of buildup, when the delicate intima cells of the artery are first roughened or invaded by oxidized LDL cholesterol or other factors, aspirin can keep platelets from collecting and clotting on the damaged area. This initial "lump" can cause a greater accumulation of the building blocks of atherosclerosis, thereby speeding the process. In short, aspirin helps keep the intimal cells smooth.

The observation that heart disease could be prevented through the use of aspirin was made more than thirty years ago by an observant practitioner in Texas who noticed that his patients with arthritis who were being treated with aspirin had much less heart disease in comparison to arthritics not receiving aspirin.

He published these mysterious results in the *Journal of the American Medical Association* and there the matter stood. Then, in 1979, a group of British researchers won the Nobel Prize for their research on prostaglandins. Among the things they found was that prostaglandins cause swelling, fever, immune reactions, headaches, menstrual cramps, and—most important for our purposes—blood clotting. One of the prostaglandins, Thromboxane A_2, swings into action when a patch of platelets are needed to stop bleeding from a wound.

The British researchers found that aspirin prevents platelets from clumping by inactivating Thromboxane A_2.

FROM PREVENTER TO LIFESAVER

The prostaglandin findings led heart researchers to several astonishing discoveries about aspirin and its role in changing the course of heart disease. Research done by M. Abramowicz and published in *Medical Letters* concludes that platelet aggregation, a major contributor to atherosclerosis, can be stopped and the clotting even reversed with the proper use of aspirin. The question was, "How much aspirin constitutes proper use?"

Researchers set out to answer that question. Charles Hennekens of Harvard University headed a study in which 22,071 healthy male physicians around the country took either an aspirin or a placebo every other day. The study showed that even such a small dose could reduce the risk of heart attack in a healthy population by 44 percent. However, the total number of deaths from all causes was the same in both groups. Although the aspirin group had less heart problems than the placebo group, the aspirin group had more strokes and stomach ulcers.

What is aspirin's effect on a not-so-healthy population? To answer that question, British researchers launched the International Study of Infarct Survival (ISIS), in which 17,000 heart-attack victims were given aspirin alone or in combination with the clot-dissolving enzyme *streptokinase*. The results showed that a combination of the two drugs could cut mortality by 50 percent if given within four hours of the onset of a heart attack. Aspirin alone reduced deaths by 20 percent when given within twenty-four hours.

Can aspirin prevent second heart attacks? Six studies involving a total of 11,000 men who had had one heart attack showed that an aspirin a day reduced their risk of another heart attack by 20 percent.

All of these studies tend to show that regular and proper use of aspirin can halt, slow, or reverse the process of atherosclerosis.

RECOMMENDATION: AN ASPIRIN (325 MILLIGRAMS) EVERY OTHER DAY

So how much aspirin should be included in the reversal diet? The research has clearly shown that an aspirin every other day provides maximum benefit with minimum risk. What is the risk? Blood that is too "thin" puts one at higher risk for stroke. As with so many other things in life and medicine, a little is good and a little more is, well, not so good.

There are other factors to keep in mind with aspirin. Since it can irritate the lining of the stomach you might want to try something besides plain aspirin. The buffered variety contains an antacid to help neutralize stomach acid. It won't protect the lining of the stomach from damage, but it will eliminate gastrointestinal pain.

Safety-coated aspirin dissolves not in the stomach but in the small intestine where it can't inflame the stomach lining. The risk of irritating the lining of the stomach or possibly causing an ulcer is not trivial.

As with any other medication, you should consult your doctor before regular aspirin use. He will want to know if you have any conditions that would prevent you from taking this most popular of drugs—maladies such as ulcers, kidney problems, gout, asthma, allergies, cancer, or any gastrointestinal bleeding. Pregnant or breast-feeding women should also consult their physician before regular aspirin use.

Keep in mind, too, that not all aspirin tablets contain the same amount of acetylsalicylic acid. Some, as you can see from the table of popular brands below, contain a much higher dose than the 325 milligrams recommended in the reversal diet.

Table 23. ASPIRIN PRODUCTS—COMPARATIVE STRENGTH

Product	Dosage/Form	Strength (mg)
Alka-Seltzer	1 tablet, effervescent	324
Ascriptin	Tablet, buffered	325
Aspergum	Chewing gum	227
Bayer	Tablet, buffered	325
Bufferin	Tablet, buffered	324
Buffinol	Tablet, buffered	324
Ecotrin	Tablet, safety coated	325
8-hour Bayer	Tablet, time released	650
Encaprin	Capsules, safety-coated granules	325, 500
Maximum Bayer	Tablet	500
Measurin	Tablet, time released	650
Norwich Aspirin	Tablet	325

THE
REVERSAL
DIET MENU

9

T he question most often asked about the reversal diet program is, "Will it leave me feeling deprived?" That is an important question, because as you probably know from personal experience, a diet that leaves you feeling hungry is one that you will likely drop in a short period of time. Eating is one of life's great pleasures, and most people aren't willing to forgo it for very long.

But the reversal diet program isn't like most other so-called diets. It is designed to help you reach your goals while you taste abundantly of life's pleasures.

To give you an idea of what the reversal diet looks like in practice, we* have assembled a week's worth of meals and their nutrient contents. This menu plan draws on the recipes that begin on page 234. It offers a wide array of foods so you can be sure there will be enjoyment in this program. Substitution is the key, not deprivation. You can have a satisfying number of calories; just make sure that the saturated-fat and cholesterol content of those calories are low.

This menu plan offers 1,500 to 2,500 calories per day, which is the usual range of caloric need. These can be adjusted to individual caloric needs by adding or subtracting snacks. If you add snacks, use one from another day. There is a substantial amount of food in these daily menu plans, yet these meals will keep you well within the reversal goals. The saturated-fat content of these meals is under the 10 percent allowed in the program, total fat is under 30 percent of total calories, and the cholesterol content of these meals never comes close to the 300 milligrams of daily intake allowed. You might say you are on a diet, but you sure can't say you're starving.

MONDAY

Breakfast

1 Oat Flake Muffin (page 309)
½ cup nonfat yogurt
1 cup strawberries
1 tsp margarine
1 tsp jam

coffee or tea
(Lighten with skim milk. Use
  artificial sweeteners if they are
  palatable.)

Lunch

cheese sandwich:
  2 slices whole-wheat bread
  1 tbsp light mayonnaise
  lettuce & tomato
  1 slice light American cheese

1 cup vegetable soup (meatless)
8 oz skim milk
1 peach (low sugar if canned
  peaches)

Dinner

1 serving Spaghetti with Meat
  Sauce (page 255)
tossed salad
2 tbsp cholesterol-free Italian
  Dressing (page 276)

8 oz skim milk
2 slices French or Italian bread
Orange Juice Yogurt Shake (page
  306)

Snack

3 cups air-popped popcorn

Nutrient values of day's meals:
Total fat calories: 260 (15%)
Saturated-fat calories: 103 (6%)
Total calories: 1,704

Cholestrol (mg): 71
Sodium (mg): 2,634

TUESDAY

Breakfast

1 toasted English muffin
¼ cantaloupe
1 cup nonfat yogurt
1 tsp margarine

1 tsp jam
8 oz skim milk
coffee or tea

Lunch

tossed salad
2 tbsp Poppy-seed Dressing (page
   277)
bowl of chicken-noodle soup
   (prepared dry variety)

10 Saltine crackers
4 oz fruit sorbet
iced tea

Dinner

1 serving Lentil and Nut Roast
   (page 286)
1 serving Green Bean Salad
   (page 267)

1 slice whole-grain bread
1 serving Apple Crisp (page 300)
8 oz skim milk

Snack

1 banana

Nutrient values of day's meals:
Total fat calories: 319 (18%)
Saturated-fat calories: 82 (4%)
Total calories: 1,824

Cholesterol (mg): 37
Sodium (mg): 2,643

WEDNESDAY

Breakfast
1 bowl oatmeal   1 tsp brown sugar
4 oz skim milk   coffee or tea
½ banana

Lunch
Submarine sandwich   1 cup tomato soup
   sub loaf of bread   1 cup grapes
   1 tbsp light mayonnaise   8 oz skim milk
   3 oz white meat turkey
   lettuce & tomato

Dinner
1 serving Orange Roughy and   2 slices French bread
   Vermicelli (page 234)   iced tea
1 serving Squash and Zucchini   1 serving Healthful Berry
   (page 274)   Shortcake (page 302)

Snack
1 apple

Nutrient values of day's meals:
Total fat calories: 229 (13%)   Cholesterol (mg): 33
Saturated-fat calories: 74 (4%)   Sodium (mg): 2,065
Total calories: 1,765

THURSDAY

Breakfast

1 toasted bagel   ½ cup nonfat yogurt
1 tbsp low-fat cream cheese   4 oz orange juice
1 tbsp jam   coffee or tea

Lunch

tossed salad   1 slice French bread
2 tbsp light Italian dressing   iced tea
1 cup tomato soup

Dinner

2 pieces mushroom pizza   8 oz skim milk
1 serving Magic Minestrone soup   1 serving Chocolate Angel Food
    (page 260)   Cake (page 299)

Snack

1 pear

Nutrient values of day's meals:
Total fat calories: 180 (9%)   Cholesterol (mg): 20
Saturated-fat calories: 60 (3%)   Sodium (mg): 3,156
Total calories: 1,804

FRIDAY

Breakfast

1 bowl of Cheerios
½ banana
4 oz skim milk

1 tsp sugar
coffee or tea

Lunch

tuna on pita-bread sandwich
    pita bread
    tuna salad made with light
      mayonnaise
    chopped tomato

1 cup tomato-rice soup
1 apple
8 oz skim milk

Dinner

1 serving Chicken and Rice
    (page 244)
1 serving Summer Squash (page
    271)

2 slices French bread
iced tea
1 serving Rice Pudding (page
    298)

Snack

3 cups air-popped popcorn

Nutrient values of day's meals:
Total fat calories: 236 (13%)
Saturated-fat calories: 58 (3%)
Total calories: 1,798

Cholesterol (mg): 92
Sodium (mg): 2,703

SATURDAY

Breakfast
1 Blueberry Muffin (page 310)   1 tsp jam
1 cup nonfat yogurt   4 oz orange juice
1 tsp margarine   coffee or tea

Lunch
Spaghetti Primavera Light (page   1 slice French bread
  250)   1 banana
Spinach Soup (page 261)   iced tea

Dinner
1 serving Salmon Oriental (page   1 dinner roll
  240)   8 oz skim milk
1 serving Sesame Noodles (page   1 serving Red Wine Pears (page
  275)   296)

Snack
1 cup nonfat frozen yogurt

Nutrient values of day's meals:
Total fat calories: 240 (12%)   Cholesterol (mg): 115
Saturated-fat calories: 77 (4%)   Sodium (mg): 2,084
Total calories: 1,887

SUNDAY

Breakfast
Fruit salad (apples, bananas, grapes, pears, pineapple in their own juices)
1 cup nonfat yogurt
1 toasted bagel
1 tbsp light cream cheese
1 tbsp jam
4 oz orange juice
coffee or tea

Lunch
1 serving Chicken Chili (page 243)
1 serving Potato Salad (page 270)
2 slices French bread
1 banana
iced tea

Dinner
1 serving Vegetable Lasagna (page 252)
tossed salad
2 tbsp Poppy Seed Dressing (page 277)
1 slice Frozen Yogurt Pie (page 294)
coffee or tea

Snack
1 pear

Nutrient values of day's meals:
Total fat calories: 310 (14%)
Saturated-fat calories: 136 (6%)
Total calories: 2,182
Cholesterol (mg): 76
Sodium (mg): 2,156

Real People, Real Meals

To show that real people do eat this way and do so without feeling deprived, I have included the actual food diaries of two of my patients.

Both of these patients had problems when they came to me. One of them had documented coronary artery disease, the other one was coronary prone.

I put these patients on the reversal diet program. That was ten years ago. Through the program presented in this book they have maintained high levels of physical fitness, achieved ideal body fat, and dropped their total cholesterol count to below 200 mg/dl while elevating their HDL cholesterol to the desired range.

They took special care in the preparation of their food at home and the selection of what they ate while at restaurants. And, as you can see from the diet diary examples shown here, no one was starving.

PATIENT ONE: AT AGE SIXTY-EIGHT, HE'S AS FIT AS A FORTY-EIGHT-YEAR-OLD

At the age of sixty-one, this patient began feeling the chest pains of angina pectoris. Angiograms showed that the left anterior descending coronary artery was 95 percent closed. He underwent balloon angioplasty, but within five months the artery had become blocked again. A third and then fourth balloon angioplasty was performed, but when the blockage recurred he decided to undergo coronary artery bypass surgery.

After surgery he was referred to me.

I prescribed a reversal diet program that included vigorous exercise and the dietary restriction of foods containing cholesterol and saturated fats.

Now, seven years after his bypass surgery, this patient's total cholesterol level has dropped from 235 mg/dl to 133 mg/dl, his ratio of HDL to total cholesterol is an incredible 2.4, and his percentage of body fat has dropped from 20 percent to 15 percent.

His exercise program has improved his functional aerobic capacity considerably. At the age of sixty-eight he runs three to five miles three times per week, rides a stationary bicycle several times per week, and walks instead of drives whenever possible.

As a result of dietary changes and a strenuous exercise program, this patient has the physical fitness of a normal forty-five year old. He has experienced no angina pains in the past six years.

Here are two days selected from a diet diary that I recently had him keep:

TUESDAY

Breakfast
½ cup oat bran
½ cup oatmeal
½ cup skim milk

2 tbsp raisins, seedless
1 medium banana, raw
3 tbsp Grape-Nuts

Morning Snack
1 cup tea, brewed

1 average water bagel

Lunch
3 oz iceberg lettuce, raw
1 oz red tomato, raw, sliced
1 oz carrots, raw
1 oz cucumber, raw
1 oz chicken fryer, dark meat
without skin
1 oz chicken fryer, light meat
without skin

2 tbsp Italian dressing
2 slices white bread, enriched
1 cup decaffeinated coffee,
instant
1 tbsp whole milk

Afternoon Snack
1 average water bagel

Dinner
6 oz Sockeye salmon, steak
½ cup long grain rice, enriched,
without salt

1 cup green beans
½ cup vanilla ice milk, soft
1 tbsp chocolate sauce

Evening Snack
½ cup orange juice

1 package unsweetened gelatin

Nutrient value of Tuesday's meals:
Total fat calories: 388 (20%)
Saturated-fat calories: 67 (4%)
Total calories: 1,854

Cholesterol (mg): 126
Sodium (mg): less than 3,300 mg

SATURDAY

Breakfast
½ cup oat bran
½ cup oatmeal
½ cup skim milk
2 tbsp raisins, seedless
1 medium banana, raw

3 tbsp Grape-Nuts
1 package unsweetened gelatin
1 cup water
1 cup coffee, brewed
1 tbsp skim milk

Lunch
½ cup lentils, boiled
½ cup water
½ cup hummus

2 slices white bread, enriched
1 cup coffee, brewed
1 tbsp skim milk

Afternoon Snack
4 oz vanilla ice milk, soft

Dinner
1 cup macaroni
¼ cup mushroom pieces, boiled,
   drained
¼ cup tomato, raw, chopped

1 cup green beans
1 average English muffin, plain
1 tbsp marmalade

Nutrient value of Saturday's meals:
Total fat calories: 212 (13%)
Saturated-fat calories: 37 (2.3%)
Total calories: 1,572

Cholesterol (mg): 211
Sodium (mg): less than 3,300 mg

PATIENT TWO: FIT ENOUGH FOR MARATHONS

At the age of fifty-seven, this patient was concerned about his heart health. He was about fifteen pounds overweight and had 22 percent body fat, far too high for a man.

That was ten years ago. Now, after a decade on the reversal diet program, his body weight has decreased twenty pounds and his percent of body fat has dropped twelve points to 10 percent.

His other numbers are very good, too. At present his total cholesterol is 206 mg/dl, with a ratio of total cholesterol to HDL of 2.7, well within the reversal range.

With a progressive program of jogging, running, and long distance running, this patient has completed six marathons.

Two days of dietary diaries were selected from a routine seven-day period to show this athlete's lowest and highest caloric intake:

MONDAY

Breakfast
½ medium banana, raw
1 tbsp bran
½ cup oat bran

1 cup oatmeal
2 oz skim milk
1 cup herb tea, brewed

Lunch
1 average water bagel
3 oz dry curd cottage cheese, unsalted, lowfat

2 oz lettuce
2 oz garbanzo beans (chickpeas)
1 medium pear

Afternoon Snack
1 large pretzel

1 medium apple

Dinner
6 oz rainbow trout fillet
4 oz potato
⅓ cup summer squash, sliced, boiled, drained
1 cup lettuce
1 tsp lemon juice, fresh

4 oz wine, 11.5% alcohol by volume
2 pieces French bread
1 cup tea, herb brewed
3 wedges cantaloupe

Evening Snack
3 oz popcorn, plain
½ oz raisins, seedless

1 large pretzel
½ grapefruit

Nutrient value of Monday's meals:
Total fat calories: 237 (11%)
Saturated fat calories: 32 (1.5%)
Total calories: 2,085

Cholesterol (mg): 131
Sodium (mg): less than 3,300 mg

TUESDAY

Breakfast
1 medium orange
½ medium banana, raw
1 tbsp brewer's yeast
1 tbsp bran
½ cup oat bran

1 cup oatmeal
2 oz skim milk
1 oz Spoon Size Shredded Wheat
1 oz raisins, seedless
1 cup herb tea, brewed

Morning Snack
1 large pretzel

Lunch
1 slice pita bread, round, whole
1.5 oz soybean curd (Tofu)
½ medium tomato
3 oz lettuce

½ tsp prepared yellow mustard,
    regular
1 cup tea, herb brewed
1 medium pear
½ medium banana, raw

Afternoon Snack
1 large pretzel

1 medium pear

Dinner
4.5 oz minestrone soup
1 oz roasted turkey, light meat
    without skin
3 pieces French bread

2 tbsp apple butter
1 medium apple
1 cup herb tea, brewed

Evening Snack
1 large pretzel
1 medium pear

3 oz popcorn, plain
1 cup herb tea, brewed

Nutrient value of Tuesday's meals:
Total fat calories: 234 (10%)
Saturated-fat calories: 32 (1.4%)
Total calories: 2,244

Cholesterol (mg): 23
Sodium (mg): less than 3,300 mg

Certainly there are more restrictive programs that one could follow. But I have found that people don't stay with the restrictive programs very long.

I have treated hundreds of patients from whom I could draw to illustrate the important points shown by these two: The reversal diet program is easy to follow for a lifetime, and the reversal diet program works.

GOOD HEALTH: Your Greatest Possession

Almost everyone who follows the reversal diet program lowers his or her cholesterol levels and reduces the risk factors that contribute to heart disease.

The National Cholesterol Education Program calls for dietary changes that are capable of lowering the cholesterol levels of an estimated 96 percent of the people who follow them. Since the reversal diet program calls for greater dietary changes than the NCEP and adds exercise, it is safe to say that at least an equal number of people will improve their total cholesterol levels and other reversal numbers by following the advice in this book.

But what if you give the reversal diet program a try and after three months you find that your cholesterol level is still higher than the numbers called for in the program? My first advice is to try again. Watch your diet even more closely. Are you still eating some foods that are high in saturated fats and cholesterol? Are you eating enough fiber, especially soluble fiber? Are you exercising enough? Are you varying from the reversal diet program in any way?

If the answer is honestly "no," you may have to see your doctor about drug treatment to lower cholesterol. Drug treatment does not replace the reversal diet program; it works with it. Returning to a high-fat diet can negate many of the benefits of drug treatment, and it can also increase your risk of other medical problems such as gallstones and colon cancer. A good diet also makes you feel better physically and mentally, because of the sense of personal control you receive from being in charge of what you eat.

CHOLESTEROL-LOWERING DRUGS

There are five classes of drugs used to lower cholesterol, each with its own benefits and side effects:

Bile-acid sequestrants: Bile-acid resins (cholestyramine and colestipol) work in the intestines to bind bile acids, which are high in
cholesterol. This forces the liver to pull more LDL cholesterol from
the bloodstream to produce bile for digestion. Bile sequestrants are
formulated as powders that dissolve in fruit juices and make for a gritty
drink. Side effects may include gas, a bloated feeling, diarrhea, or
constipation.

Fibric acids: Drugs in this class (bezafibrate, clofibrate, fenofibrate,
gemfibrozil) increase the activity of an enzyme that breaks down lipoproteins in the bloodstream and leads to a reduction of LDL and
sometimes to an increase in HDL, the protective cholesterol. Exactly
how these drugs work is unknown. Side effects may include liver
problems and gallstones.

Nicotinic acid: This oldest cholesterol-lowering drug (niacin) is
considered by many physicians to be the best. It is a vitamin that
works in the liver to decrease lipoprotein production and blood levels
of LDL. Side effects may include flushing of the skin, itching, and
stomach irritation.

Probucol: This drug alters the makeup of LDL, causing it to be
removed more quickly from the bloodstream. Probucol usually lowers
LDL cholesterol by about 15 percent but may also lower the "good"
HDL. Side effects may include abdominal pains, nausea, and diarrhea.

Enzyme inhibitors: These new cholesterol-lowering drugs inhibit
the manufacture of cholesterol by the liver. When this happens, the
liver is forced to remove LDL from the bloodstream to meet its needs.
These drugs may lower total cholesterol as much as 30 percent. Side
effects may include headache, stomach ache, rash, and an elevation
in blood levels of some liver enzymes.

SEND IT BACK

Although I recommend a nondrug approach to all my patients, I think
it is important ultimately to reach the reversal goals of this program
in any way you can in order to prevent and reverse heart disease.
Now, more than ever, it is clear to the medical world that reducing
your risk of heart disease simply means that the clogging of arteries is
stopping or being reversed.

Here is what Dr. Daniel Steinberg, a lipid scientist and member of
the NCEP's expert panel on high-blood-cholesterol treatment, said

about reversing heart disease at the 62nd Scientific Session of the American Heart Association:

> One of the things that has been demonstrated by recent studies is that the lowering of cholesterol isn't working by stopping thrombosis or preventing arrhythmias. It is working by preventing new lesions and reversing those that exist. This happens even in men who have extremely progressed lesions of the arteries.
>
> We know from studies that you can totally reverse the fatty streak lesions in animals. So these studies show us that, yes, us old characters with bad arteries will benefit even at an advanced stage. But the message is that if it [reversal] works in the older people, it will really work in the younger people.

As I've said throughout this book: heart disease can be reversed. By taking control of your life-style you can send heart disease back from where it came—you can once again have clear and healthy arteries. The reversal program isn't difficult or expensive. And the benefits are many, especially if it is started before atherosclerosis has progressed very far. After all, there is no greater possession than good health.

PART
II

RECIPES

10

FINS AND FEATHERS

When it's meat you want, most doctors and nutritionists recommend that you make it a meal from finned or feathered animals. Fish and chicken offer tasty benefits over red meats.

Fish contains Omega-3 oils that have been shown to help prevent unnecessary blood clotting and reduce blood pressure.

Chicken is beneficial to the heart because it contains much less saturated fat than red meat. Three ounces of roasted chicken breast contain 0.9 grams of saturated fat, whereas the same amount of lean, broiled sirloin steak contains 6.4 grams. With each gram of fat equaling 9 calories, the steak has almost 50 calories of saturated fat more than the chicken.

But perhaps the greatest benefit of all is the number of ways in which these finned and feathered friends can be prepared. As you can see in the following recipes, their variety can spice your life.

ORANGE ROUGHY AND VERMICELLI

SERVES FOUR

4 fresh tomatoes, peeled and cored
½ large green pepper, chopped
½ medium onion, chopped
1 clove of garlic, minced
1 teaspoon instant bouillon
1 bay leaf
¼ teaspoon thyme leaves
½ teaspoon herb seasoning, salt-free
Pinch of red pepper
1 pound orange roughy cut into 4 equal pieces
¾ pounds uncooked vermicelli pasta

Process the tomatoes in a blender until smooth. Combine tomatoes in a skillet with green pepper, onion, garlic, bouillon, bay leaf, thyme, herb seasoning and red pepper. Bring to a boil and then reduce the heat, simmering for 15 minutes. Add fish and simmer for about 10 minutes or until fish flakes when poked with a fork. Remove the bay leaf.

Prepare the vermicelli as directed on the package. Arrange on a platter and top with fish and sauce.

NUTRIENT VALUES PER SERVING

Calories: 374

Cholesterol: 68 mg

Polyunsaturated fat: 0.44 g

Saturated fat: 0.23 g

Carbohydrate: 56.5 g

Protein: 31 g

Fiber: 3.9 g

Sodium: 178 mg

SHRIMP AND SWORDFISH KABOBS

SERVES FOUR

1 tablespoon fresh lime juice
½ fresh pineapple, cut into chunky cubes, reserving the juice
4 tablespoons olive oil
2 tablespoons Worcestershire sauce
1 garlic clove, minced
½ teaspoon ground ginger
Ground black pepper to taste
1 pound swordfish steak, cut into chunky squares
½ pound shelled green shrimp
1 large green pepper, cleaned and cut into 8 pieces
12 cherry tomatoes
3 small white onions, peeled and quartered
12 mushrooms (use your favorite)

In a large bowl combine lime juice, 3 tablespoons of pineapple juice from the pineapple chunks, 2 tablespoons of olive oil, Worcestershire sauce, garlic, ginger, and black pepper (if desired). Marinate the swordfish, shrimp, vegetables, and pineapple at room temperature for 30 minutes. Remove from marinade and skewer them alternately.

Grill under broiler or on hot coals for about 5 minutes per side or until done, basting frequently with the remaining olive oil.

NUTRIENT VALUES PER SERVING

Calories: 379
Cholesterol: 133 mg
Polyunsaturated fat: 2.6 g
Saturated fat: 3.2 g

Carbohydrate: 17.8 g
Protein: 32 g
Fiber: 3.2 g
Sodium: 336 mg

BAKED SNAPPER WITH GINGER SALSA

SERVES FOUR

2 cups peeled, diced tomatoes
2 tablespoons chopped onion (white or green)
2 tablespoons chopped cilantro
2 tablespoons chopped jicama
2 tablespoons fresh lime juice
1 tablespoon minced jalapeño pepper
2 teaspoons chopped gingerroot
4 red-snapper fillets (1 pound)
1 cup dry white wine
Juice of ½ fresh lime

Salsa: Combine tomatoes, onion, cilantro, jicama, lime juice, jalapeño pepper, and gingerroot in bowl. Cover and let sit for at least one hour.

Fish: Preheat oven to 425 degrees. Place fillets in a shallow pan and cover with wine and lime juice. Cover pan with aluminum foil and bake for 25 minutes or until fish flakes when poked with a fork.

Arrange fish on a serving plate and spoon salsa on top.

NUTRIENT VALUES PER SERVING

Calories: 178
Cholesterol: 42 mg
Polyunsaturated fat: 0.61 g
Saturated fat: 0.35 g

Carbohydrate: 6.5 g
Protein: 24.3 g
Fiber: 1.7 g
Sodium: 92 mg

GRILLED SWORDFISH WITH TOMATO VINAIGRETTE

SERVES FOUR

1 pound fresh swordfish
4 tablespoons olive oil *plus additional for basting*
4 tablespoons rice vinegar
½ teaspoon dry mustard
4 scallions, chopped
½ cup fresh cilantro leaves
4 large tomatoes, chopped
Ground pepper to taste

Cut fish into four equal pieces and broil it in the oven or grill it over coals. Make certain to brush fish with olive oil to keep it moist.

Whisk oil, vinegar, and mustard. Stir in scallions, cilantro, and tomatoes. Season with pepper.

When the fish flakes when poked with a fork, arrange it on a plate and spoon vinaigrette on top.

NUTRIENT VALUES PER SERVING

Calories: 322
Cholesterol: 43 mg
Polyunsaturated fat: 2.9 g
Saturated fat: 3.3 g

Carbohydrate: 9.3 g
Protein: 28.4 g
Fiber: 3.1 g
Sodium: 59 mg

POACHED FILLET OF SOLE

SERVES FOUR

½ cup chopped onion
¼ cup chopped celery
1 tablespoon vegetable oil
4 sole fillets, skinned
1 tablespoon fresh lemon juice
1 small bay leaf
½ cup white wine
1 sprig of parsley

In a large pan, sauté the onion and celery in oil. When the vegetables are tender, place the skinned sole fillets on top of them and add the lemon juice, bay leaf, wine, and parsley. Cover and simmer at low heat for about 10 minutes or until the fish flakes when poked with a fork.

NUTRIENT VALUES PER SERVING

Calories: 163

Cholesterol: 60 mg

Polyunsaturated fat: 2.3 g

Saturated fat: 0.76 g

Carbohydrate: 2.4 g

Protein: 21.7 g

Fiber: 0.41 g

Sodium: 102 mg

MARINATED SWORDFISH STEAKS

SERVES FOUR

2 tablespoons vegetable oil
⅓ cup tarragon vinegar
1 teaspoon Worcestershire sauce
1 small bay leaf
2 tablespoons chopped parsley
Ground pepper
4 swordfish steaks, ¼ pound each

In a shallow baking pan, combine oil, vinegar, Worcestershire sauce, bay leaf, parsley, and pepper. Add the swordfish steaks, cover and refrigerate for at least 3 hours, turning the steaks to make sure they are marinated throughout. Remove the steaks from the marinade and place on a foil-covered broiler pan. Baste with marinade. Broil for about 10 minutes or until the fish flakes when poked with a fork.

NUTRIENT VALUES PER SERVING

Calories: 203
Cholesterol: 44 mg
Polyunsaturated fat: 5 g
Saturated fat: 2.1 g

Carbohydrate: 1.8 g
Protein: 22.6 g
Fiber: 0.07 g
Sodium: 126 mg

SALMON ORIENTAL

SERVES FOUR

4 salmon steaks (1¼ pounds total)
1 teaspoon sesame oil
1 teaspoon grated ginger
4 teaspoons low-sodium soy sauce

Arrange salmon on a plate. Brush sesame oil over surface and then sprinkle with ginger. Sprinkle salmon steaks with half the soy sauce, then turn them over and sprinkle with the rest of the soy sauce. Cover and refrigerate at least 30 minutes.

Heat broiler and then broil the steaks for about 10 minutes or until they are cooked to your liking.

NUTRIENT VALUES PER SERVING

Calories: 254

Cholesterol: 97 mg

Polyunsaturated fat: 3.1 g

Saturated fat: 2.2 g

Carbohydrate: 0.6 g

Protein: 30.7 g

Fiber: 0.01 g

Sodium: 416 mg

SALMON SALAD EXTRAORDINAIRE

SERVES FOUR

4 salmon steaks, 6 ounces each
1 tablespoon olive oil
1 tablespoon red wine vinegar
1 tablespoon chopped basil
½ clove garlic, minced

VINAIGRETTE:

2 tablespoons red wine vinegar
1 teaspoon minced basil
½ teaspoon minced shallot
6 tablespoons olive oil

SALAD:

8 cups torn salad greens (red leaf lettuce, endive, red cabbage)
4 red pear tomatoes, quartered
4 yellow pear tomatoes, quartered

Place salmon in a shallow dish. Whisk together the olive oil, wine vinegar, basil, and garlic and sprinkle over salmon. Cover and refrigerate for 1 hour.

Heat broiler and broil salmon for about 10 minutes or until fish flakes when poked with a fork.

Vinaigrette: Whisk vinegar, basil, and shallot in a bowl with the olive oil. Continue to whisk until smooth.

Presentation: Toss the greens and divide among four plates. Cut salmon pieces in half and place salmon on either side of the salad. Garnish each plate with four pieces of tomato (two red and two yellow). Spoon dressing onto salad.

NUTRIENT VALUES PER SERVING

Calories: 569	Carbohydrate: 16.5 g
Cholesterol: 115 mg	Protein: 40 g
Polyunsaturated fat: 5.5 g	Fiber: 6.4 g
Saturated fat: 5.8 g	Sodium: 124 mg

ORANGE ROUGHY WITH KIWI FRUIT

SERVES FOUR

4 pieces of orange roughy (1 pound)
2 tablespoons olive oil
½ tablespoon fresh tarragon
Fresh ground pepper
¼ cup fresh lemon juice
1 kiwi fruit, sliced

Pat the fish dry on a paper towel. Brush with olive oil, then sprinkle with tarragon and pepper as desired. Microwave for 4 minutes or broil on an oiled broiling rack until fish flakes when poked with a fork. Arrange fish on a plate and sprinkle with lemon juice and garnish with fruit.

NUTRIENT VALUES PER SERVING

Calories: 175

Cholesterol: 65 mg

Polyunsaturated fat: 0.8 g

Saturated fat: 1 g

Carbohydrate: 4.2 g

Protein: 21.7 g

Fiber: 0.6 g

Sodium: 78 mg

CHICKEN CHILI

SERVES TEN

2 whole chicken breasts, boiled, skinless (1 pound)
2 cups broth drained from chicken
1 tablespoon olive oil
3 large onions, chopped
3 cloves minced garlic
4 cans (16 ounces each) kidney beans, drained and rinsed
2 cups water
1 can (16 ounces) unsalted whole tomatoes, chopped
2 cans (8 ounces each) unsalted tomato sauce
2 tablespoons oregano
2 teaspoons chili powder
¼ cup lemon juice
Dash cayenne pepper
Dash ground black pepper

Simmer chicken breasts in water until tender. Remove meat from bones and cut into ¼-inch pieces.

Warm the olive oil in a skillet over moderate heat. Add the onions and garlic and cook until softened. Add to a large pot with kidney beans. Add 2 cups of water, tomatoes, tomato sauce, oregano, chili powder, lemon juice, and peppers. Add the chopped chicken breasts and stir. Cook uncovered for 15 minutes over low heat.

NUTRIENT VALUES PER SERVING

Calories: 262	Carbohydrate: 36.8 g
Cholesterol: 28 mg	Protein: 21.5 g
Polyunsaturated fat: 0.9 g	Fiber: 7.9 g
Saturated fat: 0.7 g	Sodium: 661 mg

CHICKEN AND RICE

SERVES FOUR

1 chicken bouillon cube
½ cup cornstarch
2 pounds skinless and boneless chicken breasts
2 tablespoons olive oil
2 cups chopped unsalted canned tomatoes
½ large onion, chopped
¼ cup chopped parsley
1 teaspoon salt (optional)
¼ teaspoon pepper
1 small bay leaf
½ clove garlic, minced
1¼ cups rice
¾ pound frozen peas

D issolve bouillon cube in 1 cup of boiling water. Place cornstarch in a paper bag and add one piece of chicken at a time, shaking to coat. Brown chicken in heated oil. Add tomatoes, bouillon, onion, parsley, salt (if desired), pepper, bay leaf, and garlic. Cover and simmer for 25 minutes. Add rice and cook covered for 20 minutes or until rice is done, stirring occasionally. Add peas and cook until they are tender.

NUTRIENT VALUES PER SERVING

Calories: 548	Carbohydrate: 74 g
Cholesterol: 69 mg	Protein: 36 g
Polyunsaturated fat: 1.6 g	Fiber: 5.1 g
Saturated fat: 2 g	Sodium: 438 mg

CHICKEN BREASTS WITH LEMON SAUCE

SERVES FOUR

½ clove garlic
1 pound skinless and boneless chicken breasts
2 tablespoons fresh lemon juice
½ tablespoon dill
1 tablespoon soft tub margarine
½ teaspoon grated lemon peel
Parsley
4 thin slices lemon

Rub a 9-inch baking dish with cut side of garlic, then discard. Place chicken in dish. Sprinkle with lemon juice. Sprinkle dill on each breast. Cover and bake at 350 degrees for 30 minutes or until done, basting frequently with lemon juice.

Stir margarine and grated lemon peel together in a bowl.

Transfer chicken to plates and top with the lemon sauce. Garnish chicken with parsley and lemon slices.

NUTRIENT VALUES PER SERVING

Calories: 175	Carbohydrate: 2 g
Cholesterol: 69 mg	Protein: 26.3 g
Polyunsaturated fat: 2.3 g	Fiber: 0.2 g
Saturated fat: 1.4 g	Sodium: 84 mg

CREOLE CHICKEN

SERVES FOUR

1 pound skinless and boneless chicken breasts
2 tablespoons vegetable oil
2 cups onion, chopped
2 cups sliced fresh mushrooms
2 garlic cloves, minced
1 cup chopped celery
1 tablespoon fresh oregano
1 tablespoon fresh basil
2 cups sliced green peppers
2 cups diced fresh tomatoes
1/2 cup dry white wine
2 tablespoons lemon juice
1/2 teaspoon dried red peppers
2 tablespoons fresh parsley, chopped

Simmer the chicken breasts in water until they are done. Cut them into 1/2-inch cubes and set them aside.

Heat oil in a large pan and sauté onions until they are cooked but still firm. Add mushrooms and cook over medium heat until the liquid evaporates. Add garlic, celery, and herbs and cook over medium heat for 1 minute. Add peppers and cook for 2 minutes. Stir in tomatoes and cook for about 5 minutes. Mix in wine, lemon juice, and hot peppers, and set the creole mixture aside.

Combine the chicken and creole sauce and stir them together in the large pan. Simmer for 1 minute, sprinkle with parsley and serve.

NUTRIENT VALUES PER SERVING

Calories: 139	Carbohydrate: 6.2 g
Cholesterol: 35 mg	Protein: 14.3 g
Polyunsaturated fat: 2.5 g	Fiber: 2 g
Saturated fat: 0.9 g	Sodium: 49 mg

CHICKEN BREASTS WITH ORANGE

SERVES FOUR

1 pound skinless and boneless chicken breasts
½ teaspoon paprika
1 onion, sliced
½ cup frozen orange-juice concentrate
2 tablespoons brown sugar
2 tablespoons chopped parsley
1 teaspoon low-sodium soy sauce
½ teaspoon ginger
⅓ cup water
1 teaspoon sherry

Arrange chicken breasts in a casserole and sprinkle with paprika. Cover the chicken with onion slices.

Combine juice, brown sugar, parsley, soy sauce, ginger, water, and sherry. Pour over chicken and onion. Cover and bake for about 1 hour at 350 degrees or until the chicken meat is tender when poked with a fork.

NUTRIENT VALUES PER SERVING

Calories: 239

Cholesterol: 69 mg

Polyunsaturated fat: 0.85 g

Saturated fat: 1 g

Carbohydrate: 22.8 g

Protein: 27.3 g

Fiber: 0.6 g

Sodium: 149 mg

PASTAS AND PIZZA

Pasta is a filling and complex carbohydrate dish that can be the heart's delight. Make sure, however, that the pasta you choose doesn't contain eggs or egg yolk. This type of pasta is usually announced in bold letters on the package and is to be avoided.

Many pasta and pizza dishes are "fast" foods, in that they can be prepared quickly. Keep that in mind when you are too hungry to prepare a more time-intensive meal.

But pasta and pizza are "slow" foods, too, in the way in which their complex carbohydrates release glucose into the bloodstream, preventing a rapid rise in blood-sugar levels. This makes pastas and pizza especially good for diabetics.

SPAGHETTI PRIMAVERA LIGHT

SERVES FOUR

6 ounces calorie-reduced Italian dressing
1 green pepper, chopped
1 red pepper, chopped
¾ pound yellow summer squash, sliced
1 cup mushrooms, sliced
¼ cup chopped onion
½ pound uncooked spaghetti
3 tablespoons chopped parsley

Combine all the ingredients except the parsley in a large skillet and simmer until the vegetables are as crisp as you like. Cook the spaghetti as directed on the package.

Serve vegetables over hot spaghetti sprinkled with the parsley.

NUTRIENT VALUES PER SERVING

Calories: 240

Cholesterol: 3 mg

Polyunsaturated fat: 2.9 g

Saturated fat: 0.6 g

Carbohydrate: 42.2 g

Protein: 6.7 g

Fiber: 3.8 g

Sodium: 360 mg

FRESH TOMATO CAPELLINI

SERVES FOUR

½ pound uncooked capellini pasta
2 cups peeled and finely chopped fresh tomatoes
2 tablespoons olive oil
1 teaspoon basil leaves
½ teaspoon salt (optional)
Coarse ground pepper to taste

Cook capellini as directed on the package. While pasta is steaming, combine thoroughly with remaining ingredients. Serve hot.

NUTRIENT VALUES PER SERVING

Calories: 234

Cholesterol: 0 mg

Polyunsaturated fat: 0.6 g

Saturated fat: 0.9 g

Carbohydrate: 36.6 g

Protein: 5.6 g

Fiber: 2.5 g

Sodium: 283 mg

VEGETABLE LASAGNA

SERVES FOUR

½ pound uncooked lasagna noodles
6 fresh tomatoes, peeled and cut in small pieces
1 cup grated carrots
½ cup chopped onion
2 teaspoons basil leaves
1 teaspoon salt-free herb seasoning
⅛ teaspoon pepper
2 packages frozen spinach
3 cups chopped zucchini
2 cups sliced mushrooms
8-ounce container skim-milk ricotta cheese, whipped until
    smooth
Parsley
1 cup grated skim-milk mozzarella cheese

Prepare the lasagna noodles as directed on the package. In a blender, process the tomatoes until smooth. In a saucepan combine the tomatoes, carrots, onion, and seasonings. Simmer for 20 minutes.

Spread ¾ cup of the tomato mixture in a large baking dish. Lay down one-third of the strips of lasagna and top with tomato sauce, spinach, zucchini, mushrooms, ricotta, parsley, and mozzarella. Repeat layering twice more.

Cover and bake at 350 degrees for 45 minutes. Remove from oven and let cool for 10 minutes before cutting.

NUTRIENT VALUES PER SERVING

Calories: 415	Carbohydrate: 59.1 g
Cholesterol: 34 mg	Protein: 25.6 g
Polyunsaturated fat: 0.7 g	Fiber: 10.9 g
Saturated fat: 5.7 g	Sodium: 326 mg

TOMATO PASTA

SERVES SIX

½ *pound uncooked pasta*
Olive oil
2 yellow onions, chopped
2 teaspoons minced fresh garlic
1¾ pounds tomatoes, coarsely chopped
1 can tomato paste
⅓ cup chopped basil
⅓ cup chopped parsley
1 tablespoon thyme
1 teaspoon marjoram leaves
½ teaspoon ground black pepper
⅛ teaspoon dried red pepper flakes
¾ cup tomato juice

C ook pasta according to instructions on the package. Heat olive oil in large skillet. Add onions and garlic and cook until onions are tender. Stir in remaining ingredients and simmer for about ten minutes.

NUTRIENT VALUES PER SERVING

Calories: 178

Carbohydrate: 38.2 g

Cholesterol: 0.25 mg

Protein: 6.4 g

Polyunsaturated fat: 0.27 g

Fiber: 4.8 g

Saturated fat: 0.11 g

Sodium: 144 mg

TOMATO BASIL SAUCE FOR PASTA

SERVES SIX

7 tomatoes, fresh and ripe
1 large onion, chopped
15 leaves fresh basil or 2 tablespoons dried
1 tablespoon low-sodium soy sauce

Peel tomatoes by putting them in boiling water for 2 minutes; remove and peel with knife. Chop them fine.

Sauté the onion in a very small amount of vegetable oil. Add chopped tomatoes and cook until tender.

In a blender, purée the basil with the onion-tomato mixture. Pour in a saucepan and simmer for about 15 minutes. Add soy sauce and serve over pasta.

NUTRIENT VALUES PER SERVING

Calories: 145	Carbohydrate: 30.8 g
Cholesterol: 0 mg	Protein: 5.1 g
Polyunsaturated fat: 0.14 g	Fiber: 3.4 g
Saturated fat: 0.05 g	Sodium: 185 mg

SPAGHETTI WITH MEAT SAUCE

SERVES FOUR

½ *pound very lean ground beef*
1 *onion, chopped*
2 *cloves of garlic, minced*
6 *fresh tomatoes, cut into small pieces*
½ *teaspoon salt-free herb seasoning*
½ *teaspoon sugar*
½ *teaspoon basil leaves*
¼ *cup red wine*
½ *pound uncooked spaghetti*

In a skillet combine beef, onion, and garlic and cook until beef is done. Drain fat and set aside. In a blender combine the remaining ingredients and blend at high speed for about 30 seconds. Add tomato mixture to beef and simmer for 20 minutes.

Cook pasta according to instructions on the package and serve with the sauce.

NUTRIENT VALUES PER SERVING

Calories: 200	Carbohydrate: 29.2 g
Cholesterol: 24 mg	Protein: 13.7 g
Polyunsaturated fat: 0.21 g	Fiber: 2.8 g
Saturated fat: 0.69 g	Sodium: 29 mg

PIZZA

SERVES TWELVE

When made without animal fats or saturated vegetable oils, pizza crust is an excellent complex-carbohydrate base for what goes on it. There are excellent premade pizza crusts on the market that contain no saturated fats. Or, if you are the do-it-yourself type, here is a recipe for healthful crust.

PAN PIZZA DOUGH *Makes two crusts*
3 cups unbleached flour
¾ teaspoon salt
1 teaspoon sugar
2 packages active dry yeast
1½ cups water
2 tablespoons olive oil
1 cup whole-wheat flour

In a large bowl, combine 1½ cups unbleached flour, salt, sugar, and yeast. In a small pan heat water and oil until very hot, then add to flour mix. Blend at low speed until moist and then beat for 2 minutes. Stir in whole-wheat flour and an additional ½ to 1 cup unbleached flour as needed to form a stiff dough.

On a floured countertop, spread ¼ to ½ cup flour and knead dough for 3 to 5 minutes. Place the dough in an oiled bowl and cover with a towel. Let it rise in a warm room for about 30 minutes until it is double its size.

Punch down dough to remove air bubbles. Divide dough in half. With oiled fingers, press the dough into a 12-inch round pan sprinkled with cornmeal to keep it from sticking. Form a ½-inch rim around the crust to keep the topping on the crust.

Again, let the crust rise in a warm place for about 30 minutes until it doubles in size.

Heat oven to 400 degrees and bake the crust for 8 to 10 minutes until it is lightly browned.

Then spread one of the following sauces over the crust and bake another 20 to 25 minutes.

PIZZA SAUCE *Makes 4½ cups*
1 chopped onion
6 minced garlic cloves
4 tablespoons olive oil
2 cups chopped fresh tomatoes
1 (16 ounce) can of tomato sauce
1 (12 ounce) can tomato paste
4 teaspoons oregano leaves
4 teaspoons basil leaves
½ teaspoon pepper
Mozzarella (for cheese pizza)

In a large pan, sauté onion and garlic in oil until tender. Stir in remaining ingredients and simmer for 30 minutes.

Cover each pizza crust with equal amounts of sauce and add mozzarella (½ cup per pizza) to make cheese pizza.

NUTRIENT VALUES PER SERVING

Calories: 272	Carbohydrate: 45.4 g
Cholesterol: 0 mg	Protein: 7.9 g
Polyunsaturated fat: 0.9 g	Fiber: 5.2 g
Saturated fat: 1 g	Sodium: 414 mg

Or sprinkle one or more of the following ingredients (per pizza) to make the variations found in a pizzeria:

Ingredients	Cholesterol (mg)	Fat (g)	Sodium (mg)
Fresh mushrooms (1 cup)	0	tr	3
Green pepper (1)	0	tr	2
Mozzarella cheese (3 oz)	45	15	450
Provolone cheese (3 oz)	60	24	744
Shrimp (3 oz)	128	1	1,955

PASTA FAGIOLI

SERVES FOUR

½ tablespoon olive oil
½ large onion, chopped
1 clove garlic, crushed
1 medium carrot, sliced thin
1 medium zucchini, sliced
1 teaspoon dried basil
1 teaspoon oregano
1 (16 ounce) can unsalted whole tomatoes, with liquid
1 (16 ounce) can navy beans, drained and rinsed
Pepper to taste
½ pound uncooked rigatoni

Heat the olive oil in a large pan and cook the onion and garlic until soft. Add the carrot, zucchini, basil, oregano, tomatoes with their liquid, and beans. Cook until the vegetables are tender. Season with pepper.

While the vegetables are cooking, prepare the pasta according to the instructions on the package. Spoon servings of pasta onto four plates. Then spoon the sauce on top.

NUTRIENT VALUES PER SERVING

Calories: 319	Carbohydrate: 61.2 g
Cholesterol: 0 mg	Protein: 13.3 g
Polyunsaturated fat: 0.55 g	Fiber: 8.3 g
Saturated fat: 0.36 g	Sodium: 412 mg

SOUPS, SALADS, AND SIDE DISHES

Soups, salads, and side dishes can make the meal. They can also make the meal high in cholesterol, saturated fat, and sodium if you aren't a careful cook.

Most of these recipes contain high-fiber foods such as vegetables, which leave less room for higher-calorie foods. But an added benefit is the faster transit time caused by high-fiber foods. Since they push food through the intestines faster, these foods reduce the absorption of cholesterol.

These tasty recipes add flavor to a meal without increasing those heart-harming numbers. Add a few of these to your daily diet and see that healthy living doesn't mean deprivation.

MAGIC MINESTRONE

SERVES TEN

1 tablespoon olive oil
¼ pound lean beef stew meat, cubed
½ large onion, chopped
1 clove garlic, minced
5 cups water
1 low-sodium beef bouillon cube
½ head cabbage, chopped
2 carrots, sliced
1 cup canned chick-peas, with liquid
1 cup canned kidney beans, with liquid
2 zucchini, sliced
2 fresh tomatoes, chopped
½ cup chopped parsley
½ teaspoon thyme leaves
Pepper to taste
¼ pound medium pasta shells, uncooked

In a large pot, heat the oil. Add the beef, onion, and garlic and cook until beef is barely pinkish. Add water and bouillon cube and bring the mixture to a boil. Add the cabbage, carrots, chick-peas, and kidney beans and reduce heat. Cover and simmer for 45 minutes.

Add zucchini, tomatoes, parsley, thyme, pepper, and pasta and simmer for about 10 more minutes or until pasta is tender.

NUTRIENT VALUES PER SERVING

Calories: 147
Cholesterol: 7 mg
Polyunsaturated fat: 0.43 g
Saturated fat: 0.54 g

Carbohydrate: 24 g
Protein: 7.8 g
Fiber: 5.7 g
Sodium: 184 mg

SPINACH SOUP

SERVES FOUR

1 clove garlic, chopped fine
1 teaspoon dried tarragon
1 tablespoon olive oil
1 quart canned low-sodium chicken broth
½ pound new potatoes, peeled and halved
1 pound fresh spinach, washed well
¾ cup plain nonfat yogurt
1 tablespoon lemon juice
1 teaspoon grated lemon zest

In a large saucepan, sauté garlic and tarragon in oil for a few seconds. Add the broth and bring to a boil. Add potatoes and simmer until done.

Put the potatoes and 2 cups of the liquid into a blender and blend until smooth. Pour mixture into a bowl.

Add spinach to the broth in the saucepan and simmer until almost done. Pour broth and spinach into a blender and blend until smooth. Pour that mixture into the bowl with the potato mixture.

Add the yogurt, lemon juice, and lemon zest to the blender and blend. Combine with the other two mixtures and serve cold or hot.

NUTRIENT VALUES PER SERVING

Calories: 152	Carbohydrate: 21.2 g
Cholesterol: 3 mg	Protein: 21.2 g
Polyunsaturated fat: 0.49 g	Fiber: 5.7 g
Saturated fat: 0.96 g	Sodium: 126 mg

TOMATO PEPPER SOUP

SERVES FOUR

2 tablespoons tub margarine
2 onions, diced
1 clove garlic, finely minced
1 (16 ounce) can stewed tomatoes
½ cup peeled crushed tomatoes
1 (14 ounce) can chicken broth
1 (6 ounce) can roasted red peppers, diced
Pinch of dried thyme leaves
Dash salt and pepper
¼ cup plain low-fat yogurt
½ teaspoon grated lemon zest

Melt margarine in a large pan and add onions, stirring occasionally over medium heat until soft. Add garlic and cook about 5 more minutes. Stir in stewed tomatoes with liquid, crushed tomatoes, and chicken broth, and simmer for 5 minutes over medium heat. Stir in diced peppers, thyme, salt and pepper, and simmer another 5 minutes.

In small batches pour the mixture into a food processor or blender and purée, pouring the blended portion into a large serving bowl.

Mix yogurt and lemon zest together. Ladle soup into bowls and top each serving with a dollop of the yogurt mixture.

NUTRIENT VALUES PER SERVING

Calories: 125	Carbohydrate: 14.1 g
Cholesterol: 1 mg	Protein: 3.5 g
Polyunsaturated fat: 3.4 g	Fiber: 2.4 g
Saturated fat: 1 g	Sodium: 114 mg

CHILLED ZUCCHINI-DILL SOUP

SERVES SIX

½ cup chopped onion
1 clove garlic, minced
3 zucchini, chopped
Dash of pepper
1 (16 ounce) can unsalted chicken broth
8 ounces plain nonfat yogurt
1 tablespoon dried dill weed

In a lightly oiled saucepan, sauté onions and garlic for 2 minutes. Add zucchini and pepper and sauté 3 more minutes. Add chicken broth and bring mixture to a boil. Reduce heat and simmer until zucchini is tender. Allow mixture to cool slightly and then pour into blender or food processor and process until smooth. On low speed, blend in yogurt and dill. Cover and chill before serving.

NUTRIENT VALUES PER SERVING

Calories: 55	Carbohydrate: 9.4 g
Cholesterol: 1 mg	Protein: 4.5 g
Polyunsaturated fat: 0.1 g	Fiber: 2.7 g
Saturated fat: 0.09 g	Sodium: 36 mg

BLACK BEAN SOUP

SERVES TEN

1 pound dried black beans
4 tablespoons corn oil
1½ cups chopped onions
1 cup chopped carrots
2 cloves garlic, minced
1 teaspoon ground cumin
Red pepper to taste
8 cups cold water
1 bay leaf
¼ cup dry sherry (optional)
2 tablespoons lime juice

P lace beans in a large glass bowl and soak them overnight. Drain beans and discard water. In a large pot, heat corn oil and sauté onions, carrots, garlic, cumin, and red pepper. Sauté over medium heat until onions are tender. Add beans, the 8 cups water, and bay leaf and bring mixture to a boil. Reduce heat and simmer covered for about 3 hours or until beans are tender. Stir occasionally. Remove the bay leaf and pour the mixture into a bowl.

Blend or process about 2 cups at a time until smooth. Pour mixture back into pot and bring to a boil. Add sherry and lime juice and simmer for 20 minutes, adding more water if a thinner consistency is desired.

NUTRIENT VALUES PER SERVING

Calories: 214
Cholesterol: 0 mg
Polyunsaturated fat: 3.4 g
Saturated fat: 0.8 g

Carbohydrate: 29.5 g
Protein: 10.1 g
Fiber: 5.2 g
Sodium: 8 mg

FRUIT SHELL SALAD

SERVES TEN

½ *pound uncooked pasta shells*
8 *ounces plain low-fat yogurt*
¼ *cup orange-juice concentrate*
1 *(16 ounce) can pineapple chunks, drained*
1 *large orange, peeled, seeded, and sectioned*
1 *cup seedless red grapes, halved*
1 *kiwi fruit, peeled and sliced thin*
1 *banana, sliced*
1 *apple, cored and chopped*

P repare the pasta shells as directed on the package. Drain and set
aside to cool.

In a small bowl whisk together the yogurt and the orange-juice
concentrate. In a large bowl, combine the fruit, pasta, and yogurt
dressing. Toss and serve.

NUTRIENT VALUES PER SERVING

Calories: 158

Cholesterol: 1 mg

Polyunsaturated fat: 0.07 g

Saturated fat: 0.29 g

Carbohydrate: 35.2 g

Protein: 4 g

Fiber: 2.1 g

Sodium: 18 mg

BANANA WALDORF SALAD

SERVES FOUR

2 large bananas, peeled and thinly sliced
¾ cup finely chopped celery
⅓ cup walnuts, finely chopped
⅔ cup no-cholesterol mayonnaise

Combine all the ingredients in bowl and mix together. Cover and chill in refrigerator for about 3 hours.

NUTRIENT VALUES PER SERVING

Calories: 234	Carbohydrate: 22.8 g
Cholesterol: 11 mg	Protein: 2.1 g
Polyunsaturated fat: 11 g	Fiber: 2.3 g
Saturated fat: 3.2 g	Sodium: 273 mg

GREEN BEAN SALAD

SERVES FOUR

1 pound fresh green beans cut in 3-inch lengths
¼ cup red wine vinegar
¼ cup olive oil
1 teaspoon Dijon mustard
½ cup chopped black olives
½ cup chopped green olives
3 green onions cut into finger-length strips and then cut into
*   thin strips*

Boil beans for 5 minutes and drain well.
    Combine the red wine vinegar, olive oil, and mustard and whisk well. Add beans to the mixture and stir well. Then stir in the olives and onions and serve.

NUTRIENT VALUES PER SERVING

Calories: 216

Cholesterol: 0 mg

Polyunsaturated fat: 1.6 g

Saturated fat: 2.5 g

Carbohydrate: 11.4 g

Protein: 2.9 g

Fiber: 5.6 g

Sodium: 552 mg

THAI CHICKEN SALAD

SERVES FOUR

1 pound skinless and boneless chicken breasts
6 cups romaine lettuce, hand shredded
6 green onions, white part only, chopped
¼ red onion, diced
¼ cup cilantro leaves, chopped
2 tablespoons toasted sesame seeds

DRESSING:
½ cup rice wine vinegar
¼ cup olive oil
2½ tablespoons soy sauce
Dried red pepper to taste

Broil chicken breasts for 6 to 8 minutes or until done. Remember, oil the broiling rack only lightly.

Combine the remaining ingredients (except the sesame seeds) in a large bowl and toss.

Combine dressing ingredients in a jar and shake to mix.

Arrange salad on 4 plates. Slice chicken breasts crossways in narrow strips and arrange over the greens. Pour about 1 tablespoon of dressing over each serving (there should be dressing left over) and sprinkle with sesame seeds.

NUTRIENT VALUES PER SERVING

Calories: 226
Cholesterol: 70 mg
Polyunsaturated fat: 2.1 g
Saturated fat: 1.8 g

Carbohydrate: 6 g
Protein: 29.2 g
Fiber: 2.8 g
Sodium: 229 mg

SPICY COLE SLAW

SERVES FOUR

1 pound shredded cabbage
1 onion, thinly sliced
1 cup shredded carrots
⅓ cup cider vinegar
¼ cup vegetable oil
2 tablespoons sugar
Dash salt
½ teaspoon celery seed
Dash dry mustard

Combine cabbage, onion, and carrots in a large bowl. In a small saucepan, heat the rest of the ingredients and pour over the cabbage mixture. Toss well to coat and refrigerate. Serve cold.

NUTRIENT VALUES PER SERVING

Calories: 194
Cholesterol: 0 mg
Polyunsaturated fat: 8.1 g
Saturated fat: 1.7 g

Carbohydrate: 12 g
Protein: 0 g
Fiber: 5.1 g
Sodium: 66 mg

POTATO SALAD

SERVES FIVE

⅓ cup vegetable oil
¼ cup cider vinegar
2 tablespoons dry white wine
¼ teaspoon pepper
Dash salt
1 clove garlic, minced
½ teaspoon dried rosemary
2 pounds potatoes, cubed and boiled
½ cup chopped onion
¼ cup chopped parsley

I n a large bowl whisk vegetable oil, vinegar, wine, pepper, salt, garlic, and rosemary. Add potatoes and onions. Toss and refrigerate. Add parsley and stir just before serving.

NUTRIENT VALUES PER SERVING

Calories: 296
Cholesterol: 0 mg
Polyunsaturated fat: 8.4 g
Saturated fat: 1.8 g

Carbohydrate: 38.8 g
Protein: 3.4 g
Fiber: 3.8 g
Sodium: 38 mg

SUMMER SQUASH

SERVES FOUR

1½ pounds of green and yellow summer squash
2 garlic cloves, chopped fine
½ teaspoon dried rosemary
1 tablespoon tub margarine
1 tablespoon olive oil
2 tablespoons chopped parsley
1 tablespoon lemon juice
¾ teaspoon salt-free herb seasoning
Pepper to taste

S lice the squash crosswise.
 In a large pan, sauté the garlic and rosemary in the margarine and olive oil for a few seconds. Add the squash and cook about 4 minutes, stirring constantly.

Add parsley, lemon juice, herb seasoning, and pepper. Stir and serve.

NUTRIENT VALUES PER SERVING

Calories: 93	Carbohydrate: 8.3 g
Cholesterol: 0 mg	Protein: 2.2 g
Polyunsaturated fat: 1.6 g	Fiber: 3 g
Saturated fat: 1 g	Sodium: 42 mg

HERBED SPAGHETTI

SERVES THREE

8 ounces uncooked spaghetti
2 tablespoons fresh chopped parsley
1 tablespoon tub margarine
1 tablespoon olive oil
¼ teaspoon salt-free herb seasoning
Pepper to taste

Prepare the spaghetti as directed on the package. Drain.
Combine the hot spaghetti with the other ingredients. Toss and serve.

NUTRIENT VALUES PER SERVING

Calories: 284

Cholesterol: 0 mg

Polyunsaturated fat: 1.9 g

Saturated fat: 1.2 g

Carbohydrate: 43.8 g

Protein: 6.6 g

Fiber: 1.6 g

Sodium: 52 mg

GARDEN SPAGHETTI

SERVES SIX

½ *pound uncooked spaghetti*
2 *tablespoons tub margarine*
2 *garlic cloves, minced*
2 *cups shredded carrots*
1 *medium zucchini, sliced*
½ *cup chopped onion*
1 *tablespoon Parmesan cheese*
1 *teaspoon dried dill weed*
½ *teaspoon salt-free herb seasoning*

Prepare the spaghetti as directed on the package. In a saucepan, heat the margarine and garlic. Add the carrots, zucchini, and onion and cook over medium heat until vegetables are tender. Combine spaghetti and vegetables in a bowl and toss with the Parmesan cheese, dill, and herb seasoning.

NUTRIENT VALUES PER SERVING

Calories: 172

Cholesterol: 1 mg

Polyunsaturated fat: 1.6 g

Saturated fat: 0.8 g

Carbohydrate: 28.6 g

Protein: 4.9 g

Fiber: 3.1 g

Sodium: 81 mg

SQUASH AND ZUCCHINI À LA HOT

SERVES FIVE

4 tablespoons olive oil
4 yellow squash, sliced
6 zucchini, sliced
2 small onions, chopped
1 tablespoon minced garlic
1 teaspoon finely chopped jalapeño peppers
1 bay leaf
8 plum tomatoes, cubed
1 tablespoon dried cilantro
Pepper to taste

Heat olive oil in a large pan and add squash and zucchini. Stir fry over high heat until crisp and tender. Add onions, garlic, peppers, and stir.

Add bay leaf, tomatoes, cilantro, and pepper and continue to cook over reduced heat, stirring continuously. Remove bay leaf and serve.

NUTRIENT VALUES PER SERVING

Calories: 164	Carbohydrate: 14.8 g
Cholesterol: 0 mg	Protein: 4 g
Polyunsaturated fat: 1.1 g	Fiber: 5.6 g
Saturated fat: 1.5 g	Sodium: 22 mg

SESAME NOODLES

SERVES FOUR

8 ounces uncooked linguine
2 tablespoons peanut oil
1 tablespoon lemon juice
1 tablespoon sesame seeds
1 tablespoon chopped scallions

Cook linguine according to instructions on package. Drain and put in a large bowl. Pour in peanut oil and lemon juice and toss to coat.

Toast sesame seeds in a small skillet over low heat. If needed, olive oil can be brushed on the pan. Add toasted sesame seeds to linguine and toss with scallions.

NUTRIENT VALUES PER SERVING

Calories: 231	Carbohydrate: 33.5 g
Cholesterol: 0 mg	Protein: 5.3 g
Polyunsaturated fat: 2.6 g	Fiber: 1.4 g
Saturated fat: 1.2 g	Sodium: 2 mg

CHOLESTEROL-FREE DRESSINGS

ITALIAN DRESSING

MAKES 1 CUP

⅔ cup olive oil
¼ cup red wine vinegar
1 clove garlic, minced
1 teaspoon dried oregano
Pinch dried tarragon
¼ teaspoon salad herb seasoning, salt-free
Pepper to taste

Combine ingredients in a blender and blend at medium speed for about 2 minutes.

NUTRIENT VALUES PER SERVING

Calories: 81
Cholesterol: 0 mg
Polyunsaturated fat: 0.76 g
Saturated fat: 1.2 g

Carbohydrate: 0.4 g
Protein: 0 g
Fiber: 0.02 g
Sodium: 0 mg

POPPY SEED DRESSING

MAKES 1½ CUPS

⅓ *cup white wine vinegar*
¼ *cup sugar*
2 *teaspoons minced onions*
1 *teaspoon dry mustard*
1 *cup olive oil*
4 *teaspoons poppy seeds*

I n a blender place the wine vinegar, sugar, minced onions, and dry mustard. Blend at slow speed while slowly adding the olive oil and poppy seeds. Total blending time should be about 2 minutes.

NUTRIENT VALUES PER SERVING

Calories: 107

Cholesterol: 0 mg

Polyunsaturated fat: 0.9 g

Saturated fat: 1.2 g

Carbohydrate: 6.4 g

Protein: 0.1 g

Fiber: 0.01 g

Sodium: 0 mg

VEGETARIAN ENTRÉES

It's no secret that vegetarians are healthier on the whole
than meat eaters. Much of that is due to the high-fiber,
low-cholesterol content of the foods they eat.

Meat analogues such as cottage-cheese loaf and
vegetarian meatballs are excellent sources of soluble
fiber as well as a tasty replacement for meat products.

I don't necessarily advocate vegetarian living. But
when you consider that hamburger, meat loaf, hot
dogs, ham, and luncheon meats are the five main
sources of saturated fat in our diet, an occasional
meatless but meaty meal is a good way to reduce
dietary cholesterol.

Adequate protein is the second concern of most
people about vegetarian living. But research by
Dr. Frederick Stare of Harvard University shows that
even the strictest of vegetarians—those who eat no eggs
or dairy foods—receive almost twice the RDA for
protein.

The greatest concern about vegetarian living is the
taste of the food. I think you'll find that these recipes
will put your stomach at ease.

CHEESE AND NUT PATTIES

SERVES EIGHT

½ *pound grated low-fat mozzarella cheese*
1 *large onion, chopped fine*
1 *cup ground walnuts*
7 *cups corn flakes, not crushed*
1½ *cups liquid egg substitute*
¾ *teaspoon poultry seasoning*

SAUCE:
2 *cans cream of mushroom soup*
2 *cups water*

Combine ingredients (except sauce) and mix well with spoon. Form the mixture into about 16 patties. In a large, lightly oiled pan, brown the patties and arrange them in a baking dish. Mix the mushroom soup and water in a separate bowl and pour mixture over the patties.

Bake for 1 hour at 300 degrees.

NUTRIENT VALUES PER SERVING

Calories: 371	Carbohydrate: 31.6 g
Cholesterol: 18 mg	Protein: 17.7 g
Polyunsaturated fat: 8.5 g	Fiber: 1.3 g
Saturated fat: 5.4 g	Sodium: 1,093 mg

TOMATO/CREAM CHEESE PATTIES

SERVES FOUR

4 ounces Neufchâtel cheese
¾ cup liquid egg substitute
1 cup soda-cracker crumbs
½ cup ground walnuts
1 large onion, chopped fine
1 package vegetarian broth (available at most supermarkets)
1 can tomato soup
1 cup water

Soften cheese at room temperature. Mix ingredients except the tomato soup and water together with a spoon. Form into about 12 patties. Brown patties in a large, lightly oiled skillet and arrange in a baking dish. Combine the tomato soup and water in a separate bowl and pour the mixture over the patties.

Bake at 350 degrees for 30 to 35 minutes.

NUTRIENT VALUES PER SERVING

Calories: 395	Carbohydrate: 39.9 g
Cholesterol: 3 mg	Protein: 15.3 g
Polyunsaturated fat: 2.6 g	Fiber: 2.5 g
Saturated fat: 1 g	Sodium: 731 mg

COTTAGE CHEESE LOAF

SERVES EIGHT

1 pint small-cured, dry, low-fat cottage cheese
2 packages vegetarian broth
1¼ cup liquid egg substitute
¾ cup minced pecans
½ cup skim milk
1 teaspoon melted margarine
1 large grated onion
6 ounces Special K cereal or 3 cups corn flakes

Mix ingredients well in a large bowl. Put loaf in an oiled bread pan and bake for 1 hour at 350 degrees or in a flat baking dish for 45 minutes.

NUTRIENT VALUES PER SERVING

Calories: 196   Carbohydrate: 14.5 g
Cholesterol: 3 mg   Protein: 13.5 g
Polyunsaturated fat: 2.6 g   Fiber: 1.2 g
Saturated fat: 1 g   Sodium: 199 mg

ZUCCHINI PATTIES

SERVES FOUR

1 cup coarsely grated zucchini
¼ cup liquid egg substitute
1 large grated onion
1 cup bread crumbs
½ teaspoon sage
1 tablespoon oil

Combine all the ingredients in a large bowl and mix well. Drop the mixture by large spoonfuls onto a hot, lightly oiled frying pan. Form into patties and brown on both sides.

NUTRIENT VALUES PER SERVING

Calories: 161	Carbohydrate: 22.4 g
Cholesterol: 1 mg	Protein: 6.3 g
Polyunsaturated fat: 2.6 g	Fiber: 1.7 g
Saturated fat: 0.8 g	Sodium: 215 mg

VEGETARIAN MEATBALLS AND TOMATO SAUCE

SERVES SIX

1 cup liquid egg substitute
1 cup cracker crumbs
½ cup ground nuts
1 grated onion
½ cup grated white cheese
¼ teaspoon sage
2 cans (8 ounces each) tomato sauce
2 cups water

Mix ingredients (except tomato sauce and water) in a bowl. Form mixture into balls and cook on a greased baking sheet at 350 degrees for at least 30 minutes.

Combine tomato sauce and water in a large pot and add the vegetarian meatballs to the mixture. Simmer over low heat, stirring occasionally until sauce thickens. Serve with pasta.

NUTRIENT VALUES PER SERVING

Calories: 240   Carbohydrate: 25.4 g
Cholesterol: 6 mg   Protein: 12.4 g
Polyunsaturated fat: 1.9 g   Fiber: 3.9 g
Saturated fat: 1.9 g   Sodium: 577 mg

VEGETABLE CASSEROLE

SERVES SIX

2 carrots, sliced thin
2 celery stalks, chopped
1 can mushroom soup
2 cups cooked brown rice
4 tablespoons yeast
6 large mushrooms, sliced
1 cup chopped walnuts
1 onion, chopped fine
½ cup grated low-fat white cheese
2 tablespoons wheat germ

Steam carrots and celery until soft. Combine all ingredients except cheese and wheat germ in a large bowl and spread the mixture in a greased baking dish. Sprinkle with cheese and wheat germ and bake covered at 350 degrees for 35 minutes.

NUTRIENT VALUES PER SERVING

Calories: 294

Cholesterol: 6 mg

Polyunsaturated fat: 8.5 g

Saturated fat: 2.9 g

Carbohydrate: 29.3 g

Protein: 10.4 g

Fiber: 5.4 g

Sodium: 485 mg

LENTIL AND NUT ROAST

SERVES SIX

1 cup dried lentils
½ cup ground pecans
¼ cup liquid egg substitute
1 can (12 ounces) evaporated skim milk
½ cup vegetable oil
1½ cups corn flakes
½ teaspoon sage
1 onion, chopped

Cook lentils in water to cover until tender. Combine lentils with all the other ingredients in a bowl and pour into a greased baking dish. Bake at 350 degrees for 45 minutes.

NUTRIENT VALUES PER SERVING

Calories: 423   Carbohydrate: 34.9 g
Cholesterol: 2 mg   Protein: 15.7 g
Polyunsaturated fat: 12.6 g   Fiber: 4.8 g
Saturated fat: 3 g   Sodium: 160 mg

COTTAGE CHEESE RICE LOAF

SERVES SIX

2 cups cooked brown rice
2 cups low-fat cottage cheese
1 cup finely ground pecans
1 onion, finely chopped
¾ cup liquid egg substitute
½ teaspoon sage
2 tablespoons low-sodium soy sauce
⅓ cup evaporated skim milk

SAUCE:
1 tablespoon catsup
1 tablespoon water
½ tablespoon brown sugar

Mix the ingredients (but not those for the sauce) in a large bowl and then pour the mixture into an oiled loaf pan. Combine the catsup, water, and brown sugar into a paste and spread it over the loaf before baking. Bake at 350 degrees for 50 minutes.

NUTRIENT VALUES PER SERVING

Calories: 320	Carbohydrate: 25.9 g
Cholesterol: 7 mg	Protein: 18.7 g
Polyunsaturated fat: 3.8 g	Fiber: 2.4 g
Saturated fat: 2.2 g	Sodium: 747 mg

PECAN MEAL PATTIES

SERVES FOUR

¾ cup liquid egg substitute
1 cup grated low-fat white cheese
½ cup very finely ground pecans
¾ cup homemade bread crumbs
1 onion, finely chopped
1½ tablespoons parsley flakes
½ teaspoon garlic powder
1 package vegetarian broth
½ teaspoon oregano
1 can mushroom soup

Combine all the ingredients (except mushroom soup) in a large bowl and form mixture into small patties. Brown them quickly in a lightly oiled skillet and arrange in a baking dish. Cover with mushroom soup and bake at 350 degrees for 30 minutes.

NUTRIENT VALUES PER SERVING

Calories: 375   Carbohydrate: 25.9 g
Cholesterol: 18 mg   Protein: 17.7 g
Polyunsaturated fat: 6.3 g   Fiber: 2 g
Saturated fat: 5.7 g   Sodium: 972 mg

VEGETARIAN SAUCES

These sauces go with the "dry" dishes such as cereal loaf to make them moist and more flavorful.

BROWN GRAVY

SERVES 4

½ cup flour
2 cups cold water
¼ teaspoon onion powder
1 teaspoon dehydrated onion
2 teaspoons low-sodium soy sauce
Dash each:
    Garlic salt
    Celery salt
    Salt

Blend flour and water together until smooth. Cook this mixture over low heat and add the remaining ingredients. Cook slowly for about 10 minutes, adding water if gravy becomes too thick.

NUTRIENT VALUES PER SERVING

Calories: 56	Carbohydrate: 11.7 g
Cholesterol: 0 mg	Protein: 1.7 g
Polyunsaturated fat: 0.003 g	Fiber: 0.38 g
Saturated fat: 0.001 g	Sodium: 208 mg

MOCK CHICKEN GRAVY

SERVES EIGHT

¼ cup flour
1½ cups water
¼ teaspoon paprika
½ teaspoon dehydrated onion
1½ teaspoons vegetarian chicken seasoning

Brown the flour in a skillet and combine in a blender with all the other ingredients. Blend at high speed until mixture is smooth. Then cook until thickened.

NUTRIENT VALUES PER SERVING

Calories: 14   Carbohydrate: 3 g
Cholesterol: 0 mg   Protein: 0.4 g
Polyunsaturated fat: trace   Fiber: trace
Saturated fat: trace   Sodium: trace

VEGETABLE GRAVY

SERVES EIGHT

3 cups water
½ potato
½ onion
½ stalk celery
2 tablespoons low-sodium soy sauce
Dash each:
  Sage
  Thyme
  Garlic powder

I n a medium saucepan, combine all the ingredients and cook until vegetables are done. Then pour into a blender and blend at high speed until smooth. Simmer over low heat until gravy reaches desired thickness.

NUTRIENT VALUES PER SERVING

Calories: 12

Carbohydrate: 1.2 g

Cholesterol: 0 mg

Protein: 0.2 g

Polyunsaturated fat: trace

Fiber: trace

Saturated fat: trace

Sodium: 130 mg

DANDY DESSERTS

Many—myself included—feel that no meal is complete without dessert. Just so you know that you can have your cake and reversal too, I have included several dessert recipes that will satisfy that sweet tooth without adding fats and cholesterol.

FROZEN YOGURT PIE

MAKES ONE 9-INCH PIE, SERVES EIGHT

CRUST:

1 cup quick-cooking oats, uncooked
⅓ cup toasted wheat germ
¼ cup brown sugar
3 tablespoons tub margarine, melted
½ teaspoon cinnamon

FILLING:

1 pint frozen low-fat strawberry yogurt
1 pint frozen low-fat vanilla yogurt
1 pint strawberries, sliced thin

To make the crust, preheat oven to 375 degrees. Lightly coat a 9-inch pie pan with vegetable oil.

Combine all the ingredients for crust in a mixing bowl. Then press with your fingers into the pan. Bake for 8 to 10 minutes until crust is golden brown. Cool it completely.

For the filling, put frozen yogurts in one bowl and stir them until they are soft, almost like a thick milk shake. Then spoon the mixture into the pie shell, smoothing it as you go. When the shell is filled, freeze the pie until it is firm. Serve with berries on top.

NUTRIENT VALUES PER SERVING

Calories: 238
Cholesterol: 5 mg
Polyunsaturated fat: 2.4 g
Saturated fat: 1.7 g
Carbohydrate: 37.2 g
Protein: 8.5 g
Fiber: 2.2 g
Sodium: 129 mg

WHITE CAKE

MAKES ONE, DOUBLE-LAYER, 8-INCH CAKE

2 cups sifted cake flour
1 cup sugar
¼ teaspoon salt
1 teaspoon baking powder
⅔ cup skim milk
1 teaspoon vanilla extract
⅜ cup corn oil
6 egg whites

Preheat oven to 350 degrees. Lightly oil the bottom of two cake pans with vegetable oil. Sift the flour with the sugar, salt, and baking powder. Mix skim milk, vanilla, and corn oil in a separate bowl. Add the milk mixture to the flour mixture and beat at low speed until smooth. Beat the egg whites until stiff and fold in. Pour the batter into the cake pans and bake for 30 to 35 minutes. Cool before removing from pans.

NUTRIENT VALUES PER SERVING

Calories: 300

Cholesterol: 0 mg

Polyunsaturated fat: 4.1 g

Saturated fat: 0.89 g

Carbohydrate: 55.3 g

Protein: 4.9 g

Fiber: 3.1 g

Sodium: 120 mg

RED WINE PEARS

SERVES FOUR

2 large cans low-calorie pear halves
1 cup red wine
½ tablespoon orange zest (grated orange peel)
½ teaspoon vanilla extract

Drain pear juice into a saucepan, add wine, and cook over medium heat until mixture is reduced to a syrupy consistency.

Put pears in a large bowl and add orange zest and vanilla. Then cover with hot syrup and stir gently to combine ingredients. Refrigerate and serve cold.

NUTRIENT VALUES PER SERVING

Calories: 163   Carbohydrate: 33.5 g
Cholesterol: 0 mg   Protein: 0.9 g
Polyunsaturated fat: 0.02 g   Fiber: 8.3 g
Saturated fat: 0.008 g   Sodium: 11 mg

ICY FRUIT SMOOTHIE

SERVES FOUR

2 cups frozen strawberries
2 bananas
1 tablespoon sugar
1 cup skim milk, very cold

Combine strawberries, bananas, and sugar in a blender and begin mixing. Slowly add milk. Blend until slushy. Serve immediately.

NUTRIENT VALUES PER SERVING

Calories: 208

Cholesterol: 1 mg

Polyunsaturated fat: 0.13 g

Saturated fat: 0.18 g

Carbohydrate: 52.4 g

Protein: 3.4 g

Fiber: 3.5 g

Sodium: 36 mg

RICE PUDDING

SERVES EIGHT

1½ cups cooked rice
½ cup liquid egg substitute
3 cups skim milk
1 teaspoon vanilla
¼ cup sugar
1 teaspoon cinnamon

Spray shallow baking pan with nonstick product such as PAM. Mix all of the above ingredients and pour into shallow 9- × 13-inch baking pan. Bake at 350 degrees for 1 hour or until firm but moist. Sprinkle with cinnamon.

NUTRIENT VALUES PER SERVING

Calories: 112
Cholesterol: 2 mg
Polyunsaturated fat: 0.25 g
Saturated fat: 0.21 g

Carbohydrate: 20 g
Protein: 5.8 g
Fiber: 0.07 g
Sodium: 75 mg

CHOCOLATE ANGEL FOOD CAKE

SERVES TWELVE

1 cup plus 2 tablespoons cake flour
¼ teaspoon salt
¼ cup cocoa powder
1¼ cups sugar
12 egg whites, at room temperature
1 tablespoon lemon juice
1 tablespoon water
1 teaspoon cream of tartar
1 teaspoon vanilla extract
1 teaspoon almond extract

Preheat oven to 350 degrees. Sift flour, salt, cocoa, and half the sugar. In another bowl beat egg whites, lemon juice, water, and cream of tartar until fluffy. Add the remaining sugar, vanilla, and almond extract until mixture becomes stiff. Sift cocoa over egg whites and fold until well mixed. Pour batter into ungreased 10-inch tube pan. Bake on bottom shelf for 45 minutes. Cake should spring back when touched. Turn tube pan upside down to cool. Cake will loosen from pan. Serve angel food cake plain or with light dusting of sifted confectioners' sugar.

NUTRIENT VALUES PER SERVING

Calories: 142
Cholesterol: 0 mg
Polyunsaturated fat: 0 g
Saturated fat: 0.30 g

Carbohydrate: 29.9 g
Protein: 4.9 g
Fiber: 1.1 g
Sodium: 97 mg

APPLE CRISP

SERVES TEN

1 can (12 ounces) frozen apple-juice concentrate
2 tablespoons cornstarch
6 cups peeled and sliced tart green apples
1 tablespoon lemon juice
1 teaspoon cinnamon

Thaw apple-juice concentrate and dissolve cornstarch in it. Add sliced apples to the apple juice and cook 1 to 2 minutes, then add lemon juice. Stir and let cool.

TOPPING

1½ cups rolled oats
¼ cup wheat germ
¼ cup soft unsalted margarine
¼ cup brown sugar
2 tablespoons flour

Mix topping ingredients together until crumbly. Pour apple mixture into shallow 9- × 13-inch baking dish and sprinkle cinnamon over top. Add topping and bake at 350 degrees for 30 to 45 minutes until lightly brown on top. Serve warm.

NUTRIENT VALUES PER SERVING

Calories: 233
Cholesterol: 0 mg
Polyunsaturated fat: 1.8 g
Saturated fat: 1 g

Carbohydrate: 44.3 g
Protein: 2.8 g
Fiber: 3.4 g
Sodium: 7 mg

QUICK CHOCOLATE CAKE

SERVES NINE

1 cup sugar
1½ cups flour
¼ cup cocoa
1 teaspoon baking soda
¼ teaspoon salt
1 tablespoon lemon juice
⅓ cup vegetable oil
1 teaspoon vanilla
1 cup cold water

Mix ingredients in the order given. Pour batter into ungreased 9-inch square baking pan. Bake at 350 degrees for about 30 minutes. This is a very moist, chocolaty cake, which can be served plain or with a dusting of sifted confectioners' sugar.

NUTRIENT VALUES PER SERVING

Calories: 234   Carbohydrate: 37.6 g
Cholesterol: 0 mg   Protein: 2.5 g
Polyunsaturated fat: 4.6 g   Fiber: 1.5 g
Saturated fat: 1.4 g   Sodium: 187 mg

HEALTHFUL BERRY SHORTCAKE

SERVES EIGHT

2 cups whole-wheat flour (or 1 cup unbleached and 1 cup
    whole wheat for a lighter shortcake)
1 tablespoon baking powder
2 tablespoons sugar
1 teaspoon cinnamon
⅓ cup vegetable oil
⅔ cup skim milk
1 quart frozen low-fat vanilla yogurt
1 pint fresh blueberries
1 pint fresh strawberries

Preheat oven to 450 degrees. Mix dry ingredients (except sugar and cinnamon) in a mixing bowl. Add oil and milk to dry mixture until dough can be formed into a ball. Drop dough by tablespoons onto an ungreased cookie sheet. Sprinkle with a mixture of the sugar and cinnamon for topping. Bake approximately 12 minutes until shortcakes are golden brown.

Serve with frozen low-fat vanilla yogurt and fresh strawberries and blueberries.

NUTRIENT VALUES PER SERVING

Calories: 329

Cholesterol: 6 mg

Polyunsaturated fat: 5.6 g

Saturated fat: 2 g

Carbohydrate: 49.3 g

Protein: 10.8 g

Fiber: 5.4 g

Sodium: 237 mg

CARROT CAKE

SERVES TWELVE

2 cups sifted whole-wheat flour
2 teaspoons baking soda
½ teaspoon salt
¾ cup liquid egg substitute
¾ cup vegetable oil
¾ cup plain yogurt
1½ cups brown sugar
2 teaspoons vanilla extract
1 (8 ounce) can crushed pineapple
2 cups grated raw carrots
1 cup chopped nuts

Sift first three ingredients. Beat egg substitute, oil, yogurt, sugar, and vanilla until mixed and add to dry ingredients. Drain pineapple and combine with carrots and nuts. Blend into batter. Pour into lightly greased and floured 9- × 12- × 2-inch baking pan. Bake in 350-degree oven for 55 minutes.

NUTRIENT VALUES PER SERVING

Calories: 402

Cholesterol: 1 mg

Polyunsaturated fat: 9.6 g

Saturated fat: 2.7 g

Carbohydrate: 50.9 g

Protein: 7.4 g

Fiber: 3.9 g

Sodium: 333 mg

CARROT CAKE FROSTING

3 ounces low-fat cream cheese
¼ cup skim milk
1 teaspoon vanilla
1½ cups sifted confectioners' sugar

Blend cream cheese and milk until smooth; add vanilla and sugar. Frost when cake is cool.

NUTRIENT VALUES PER SERVING

Calories: 89

Cholesterol: 8 mg

Polyunsaturated fat: 0.09 g

Saturated fat: 1.5 g

Carbohydrate: 16.5 g

Protein: 0.7 g

Fiber: 0 g

Sodium: 24 mg

PUMPKIN SPICE BRAN CAKE

SERVES SIXTEEN

2 cups sifted unbleached flour
2 teaspoons baking powder
1 teaspoon baking soda
½ teaspoon salt
1½ teaspoons cinnamon
½ teaspoon ground cloves
¼ teaspoon allspice
¼ teaspoon ginger
2 cups sugar
1 cup liquid egg substitute
2 cups pumpkin (one 16 ounce can)
1 cup vegetable oil
1 cup 100% bran cereal
1 cup golden raisins

Preheat oven to 350 degrees. Mix all ingredients in order given. Bake in lightly greased bundt pan for 1 hour. Let cake cool. Turn cake over onto serving platter. Optional topping is sifted confectioners' sugar. This is a spicy, dense, wonderful cake.

NUTRIENT VALUES PER SERVING

Calories: 332   Carbohydrate: 47.9 g
Cholesterol: 0 mg   Protein: 4.7 g
Polyunsaturated fat: 1.8 g   Fiber: 2.7 g
Saturated fat: 1.7 g   Sodium: 219 mg

ORANGE JUICE YOGURT SHAKE

SERVES TWO

1 cup vanilla frozen yogurt
1 cup orange juice
1 cup crushed ice

Place frozen yogurt and orange juice in blender and process about 10 seconds. Add crushed ice and blend about 30 seconds until mixture is smooth but not watery. Serve immediately.

NUTRIENT VALUES PER SERVING

Calories: 208

Cholesterol: 0 mg

Polyunsaturated fat: 0.01 g

Saturated fat: 0.008 g

Carbohydrate: 40.8 g

Protein: 3.8 g

Fiber: 0.12 g

Sodium: 2 mg

MUFFINS AND BREADS

The words "oat bran" are spoken with a reverence among those who are trying to lower cholesterol levels. In many ways it is a miracle food with the almost magical ability to absorb fats and cholesterol in the digestive tract and flush them from the body before they have a chance to be absorbed into the bloodstream.

Research shows that the daily addition of oat bran and other foods with soluble fiber, such as many vegetables and fruits, can lower your cholesterol count without lowering the amount of HDL or "good" cholesterol that prevents plaque buildup on artery walls.

Insoluble fibers—the type that add bulk but don't digest—have great health benefit, too. Dr. Denis Burkitt, the fiber expert whose work is quoted in this book, feels that eating four to six slices of fibrous bread per day provides the fiber we need to lower our risk of atherosclerosis and many other diseases associated with the Western diet.

The muffin and bread recipes in this section are filled with soluble and insoluble fibers. And best of all, they are tasty.

WHOLE-WHEAT MUFFINS

MAKES 1½ DOZEN

1 cup whole-wheat flour
1 cup unbleached flour
4 teaspoons baking powder
¾ cup light brown sugar
¾ cup light raisins
4 egg whites (or ½ cup liquid egg substitute)
1 cup skim milk
⅔ cup soft margarine

In a large mixing bowl combine dry ingredients, then add sugar and raisins. In a small mixing bowl beat egg whites (or egg substitute) until foamy, and blend in milk and soft margarine. Fold milk mixture into dry ingredients just enough to moisten. Do not beat, as overmixing creates heavy, flat muffins. Spoon batter into muffin-tin liners that are lightly greased with tub margarine. Bake in preheated oven at 425 degrees for 15 to 20 minutes or until the muffins are lightly browned.

NUTRIENT VALUES PER SERVING

Calories: 169

Cholesterol: 0 mg

Polyunsaturated fat: 3 g

Saturated fat: 1 g

Carbohydrate: 25 g

Protein: 3.1 g

Fiber: 1.5 g

Sodium: 198 mg

OAT FLAKE MUFFINS

MAKES 1 DOZEN

2 cups oatmeal
¾ cup skim milk
⅓ cup vegetable oil
2 egg whites (or ¼ cup liquid egg substitute)
1½ cups unbleached flour
½ cup sugar
1 tablespoon baking powder

Preheat oven to 400 degrees. Combine cereal and milk and let stand just until softened. Add oil and egg whites (or egg substitute). Mix well. Add combined remaining ingredients, mixing until dry ingredients are just moist. Batter will be stiff. Do not overmix, or muffins will be heavy and flat. Fill one dozen lightly greased muffin tins half full. Bake at 400 degrees for 20 minutes.

Muffins should be golden brown, and toothpick inserted in center should come out clean. Let muffins cool 5 minutes before removing them from pan.

NUTRIENT VALUES PER SERVING

Calories: 198
Cholesterol: 0 mg
Polyunsaturated fat: 4 g
Saturated fat: 1 g

Carbohydrate: 29 g
Protein: 5 g
Fiber: 2 g
Sodium: 116 mg

BLUEBERRY WHEAT GERM MUFFINS

MAKES 1 DOZEN

½ cup oil
½ cup sugar
½ cup orange juice
2 egg whites (or ¼ cup liquid egg substitute)
2 cups unbleached flour
2 teaspoons baking powder
¼ teaspoon soda
¼ cup wheat germ
1 teaspoon grated orange rind
1 cup fresh or frozen blueberries

Beat oil, sugar, orange juice, and egg whites (or egg substitute). Sift dry ingredients and place in a large mixing bowl with wheat germ, orange rind, and blueberries. Combine dry ingredients with liquid mixture. Do not overmix. Bake in muffin tins for 20 minutes in 400-degree oven or until lightly browned.

NUTRIENT VALUES PER SERVING

Calories: 201
Cholesterol: 0 mg
Polyunsaturated fat: 5 g
Saturated fat: 1 g

Carbohydrate: 26 g
Protein: 9 g
Fiber: 1 g
Sodium: 99 mg

CRANBERRY OATMEAL MUFFINS

MAKES 1 DOZEN

8 tablespoons jellied cranberry sauce
1 cup quick oats
1 cup skim milk
1 cup unbleached flour
½ cup brown sugar
2 teaspoons baking powder
¼ cup soft margarine
2 egg whites (or ¼ cup liquid egg substitute)
1 tablespoon vegetable oil

Prepare muffin cups by spraying with nonstick product. Spread heaping teaspoon of cranberry sauce in bottom of muffin cups. In another bowl combine oats and milk and let stand 5 minutes. Mix flour, sugar, and baking powder. Add soft margarine, egg whites (or egg substitute), and vegetable oil to oat mixture. Beat well. Add dry ingredients to liquid mixture. Stir just until moistened. Fill prepared muffin cups ⅔ full and bake at 400 degrees for 20 minutes or until lightly browned. Serve warm.

NUTRIENT VALUES PER SERVING

Calories: 167
Cholesterol: 0 mg
Polyunsaturated fat: 2.4 g
Saturated fat: 1 g

Carbohydrate: 26.6 g
Protein: 3.4 g
Fiber: 1.1 g
Sodium: 141 mg

ORANGE MUFFINS

MAKES 18

1½ cups sugar
¾ cup soft margarine
½ cup fresh orange juice
3 teaspoons grated orange peel
3 egg whites
3 tablespoons vegetable oil
2½ cups unbleached flour
2 teaspoons baking powder

Beat sugar and soft margarine until light and fluffy. Add orange juice, orange peel, egg whites (or egg substitute), and vegetable oil. Blend well. Add dry ingredients to liquid mixture. Stir just until well moistened. Do not overmix. Line muffin cups with paper liners and fill ⅔ full. Bake at 400 degrees for about 20 minutes or until toothpick inserted in center comes out clean.

NUTRIENT VALUES PER SERVING

Calories: 157   Carbohydrate: 29.1 g
Cholesterol: 0 mg   Protein: 2.4 g
Polyunsaturated fat: 4.4 g   Fiber: 0.5 g
Saturated fat: 1.5 g   Sodium: 152 mg

BRAN MOLASSES MUFFINS

MAKES 1½ DOZEN

2 cups All-Bran cereal
1½ cups skim milk
¼ cup molasses
⅓ cup soft margarine
2 egg whites (or ¼ cup liquid egg substitute)
1½ cups unbleached flour
½ cup sugar
1½ teaspoons baking soda
½ cup raisins (optional)

Combine cereal, milk, and molasses and let stand until cereal is softened. Add soft margarine and egg whites (or egg substitute). Beat well. Combine dry ingredients in another bowl and mix well. Stir in raisins. Add cereal mixture to dry ingredients and stir just until all are moistened.

Fill lightly greased muffin cups ½ full. Bake at 400 degrees about 15 minutes or until toothpick inserted in center comes out clean. Remove from pan immediately.

NUTRIENT VALUES PER SERVING

Calories: 140
Carbohydrate: 27.1 g
Cholesterol: 0 mg
Protein: 3.4 g
Polyunsaturated fat: 1.4 g
Fiber: 3.4 g
Saturated fat: 0.5 g
Sodium: 243 mg

PUMPKIN BREAD

MAKES TWO LOAVES

3 cups sugar
1 cup vegetable oil
4 egg whites and 2 tablespoons vegetable oil (or ½ cup
   liquid egg substitute)
⅔ cup water
3½ cups unbleached flour
2 teaspoons baking soda
1 teaspoon cinnamon
1 teaspoon nutmeg
1 teaspoon allspice
2 cups (one 24 ounce can) pumpkin
1 cup chopped nuts (optional)
1 cup chopped dates (optional)

Mix sugar, oil, egg whites and vegetable oil (or egg substitute), and water. Combine dry ingredients and add to liquid. Then add pumpkin. Nuts or dates can be added if desired. Bake for 1 hour at 350 degrees. Cool for 30 minutes.

NUTRIENT VALUES PER SERVING

Calories: 194

Carbohydrate: 29.7 g

Cholesterol: 0 mg

Protein: 2.2 g

Polyunsaturated fat: 4.7 g

Fiber: 1 g

Saturated fat: 1 g

Sodium: 70 mg

CRANBERRY NUT BREAD

MAKES TWO SMALL LOAVES OR 1 DOZEN MUFFINS

2 cups flour
1 cup sugar
1 ½ teaspoons baking powder
1 teaspoon salt
½ teaspoon baking soda
¼ cup soft margarine
2 egg whites (or ¼ cup liquid egg substitute)
¾ cup orange juice
1 ½ cups chopped cranberries
1 cup chopped nuts
1 ½ cups dried currants or light raisins
1 teaspoon grated orange peel

Mix all dry ingredients in mixing bowl. Blend softened margarine into dry ingredients. Add egg whites (or egg substitute) and orange juice.

Chop cranberries and nuts in blender and add to dough along with currants or raisins and orange peel. Mix well. Bake in muffin tins or two small loaf pans lightly greased with tub margarine. Bake loaves at 350 degrees for about 50 minutes. Bake muffins at 350 degrees for about 20 minutes or until lightly browned and a toothpick inserted in the center comes out clean. Cool for 5 minutes before removing muffins from tins.

NUTRIENT VALUES PER SERVING

Calories: 190
Cholesterol: 0 mg
Polyunsaturated fat: 3.2 g
Saturated fat: 1 g

Carbohydrate: 32.5 g
Protein: 3.1 g
Fiber: 1.7 g
Sodium: 105 mg

SWEET POTATO BREAD

MAKES ONE LOAF

1 cup cooked and mashed sweet potatoes
¾ cup evaporated skimmed milk
⅓ cup frozen apple-juice concentrate
1 teaspoon low-sodium soy sauce
1 tablespoon cinnamon
¼ teaspoon nutmeg
1 envelope active dry yeast (dissolved in ½ cup lukewarm
     water)
4 cups whole-wheat pastry flour
1 tablespoon nonfat milk

Blend potatoes, evaporated milk, apple juice, soy sauce, and
spices in a food processor or blender. Transfer mixture to a large
bowl and stir in the dissolved yeast. Slowly add 3¼ cups of the flour,
stirring well to combine. Knead for 3 to 5 minutes, gradually adding
the rest of the flour. Shape the sticky dough into a loaf and place in a
lightly greased pan. Set the pan in a warm place. Let dough rise one
hour.

Preheat oven to 425 degrees and bake loaf for 10 minutes. Prick
the surface with a fork in several places and brush bread with milk.
Then turn the heat down to 375 degrees and continue baking for 35
to 40 minutes. Remove the bread from the oven and let it cool before
slicing.

NUTRIENT VALUES PER SERVING

Calories: 117	Carbohydrate: 24.7 g
Cholesterol: 0 mg	Protein: 4.8 g
Polyunsaturated fat: 0.3 g	Fiber: 3.9 g
Saturated fat: 0.02 g	Sodium: 35 mg

ZERO-CHOLESTEROL SHOPPING LIST

11

T o help you shop for the right stuff, we have included a shopping
    list of brand-name, zero-cholesterol foods.

Although these foods contain no cholesterol, some do contain a
certain amount of fat. 'In most cases, information as to the type of fat
(saturated or unsaturated) was not available. In many other cases, it
could not be accurately measured because food manufacturers often
switch between saturated and unsaturated oils depending upon avail-
ability and price.

You can avoid the small amount of saturated fat that might be
contained in these foods by refusing to buy those whose labels list
tropical oils: palm, palm kernel, or coconut.

The following list consists of commercially prepared products and
represents only a small number of the foods in each category that
contain no cholesterol. There are many others not listed here because
they have a higher fat content than the same food listed or simply
because we don't know about them.

There are also dozens of natural foods that are free of cholesterol
and saturated fats. All vegetables, for example, are "worry free" foods
that contain no cholesterol and have the added bonus of containing
very little fat of any kind. Fruit is in the same category; there is no
cholesterol in the whole lot.

So feel free to eat all the natural fare you can. But in the modern
world, it's nice to know who your brand-name friends are, too.

Table 24.   ZERO-CHOLESTEROL PRODUCTS

Brand Name	Portion	Calories	Sodium (mg)	Fat (g)	Choles. (mg)
COFFEE					
Kava					
Instant Coffee	1 tsp	2	5	0	0
Postum					
Instant Coffee	6 fl oz	11	3	0	0
FRUIT/VEGETABLE JUICES					
Bel Normande					
Apple Cider	6 fl oz	80	0	0	0
Campbell's					
V-8 Lo Sodium Vegetable Juice Cocktail	6 fl oz	40	45	0	0
V-8 Spicy Hot Vegetable Juice Cocktail	6 fl oz	35	600	0	0
V-8 Vegetable Juice Cocktail	6 fl oz	35	600	0	0
Del Monte					
Tomato Juice	½ cup	70	10	0	0
Unsweetened Pineapple Juice	6 fl oz	100	10	0	0
Unsweetened Prune Juice	6 fl oz	120	10	0	0
Dole					
Frozen Pineapple Juice	6 fl oz	90	5	0	0
Frozen Pineapple Orange Juice	6 fl oz	90	10	0	0
Frozen Pineapple Pink Grapefruit Juice	6 fl oz	101	20	0	0
Pineapple Juice	6 fl oz	100	10	0	0
Unsweetened Pineapple Juice	6 fl oz	100	10	0	0
Pineapple Grapefruit Juice	6 fl oz	90	25	0	0
Pineapple Orange Juice	6 fl oz	90	20	0	0
Pineapple/Orange/Banana Juice	6 fl oz	90	5	0	0
Hollywood					
Carrot Juice	6 fl oz	70	200	0	0
Hunt's					
Tomato Juice No Salt Added	6 fl oz	30	30	0	0
Knudsen Family					
Just Cranberry Juice	8 fl oz	40	—	0	0
Very Veggie Juice	8 fl oz	40	580	0	0
Martinelli's					
Gold Medal Apple Cider	6 fl oz	100	4	0	0
Gold Medal Apple Juice	6 fl oz	100	4	0	0

Brand Name	Portion	Calories	Sodium (mg)	Fat (g)	Choles. (mg)
Martinelli's cont.					
Gold Medal Sparkling Cider	6 fl oz	100	4	0	0
Sparkling Apple Cranberry Juice	6 fl oz	90	7	0	0
Mott's					
Apple Juice	8.45 fl oz	124	20	0	0
Apple Raspberry Juice	8.45 fl oz	120	65	0	0
Clamato Juice	6 fl oz	90	800	0	0
Country Style Prune Juice	6 fl oz	129	7	0	0
Unsweetened Prune Juice	6 fl oz	130	10	0	0
100% Pure Apple Juice—clear	6 fl oz	80	13	0	0
Ocean Spray					
Apple Juice from concentrate	6 fl oz	90	15	0	0
Unsweetened Apple Juice	6 fl oz	90	15	0	0
Unsweetened Grapefruit Juice from concentrate	6 fl oz	70	10	0	0
White Grapefruit Juice from concentrate	6 fl oz	70	10	0	0
ReaLemon					
Lemon Juice	2 tbsp	6	10	0	0
ReaLime					
Lime Juice	2 tbsp	4	10	0	0
Seneca					
Apple Juice	6 fl oz	90	20	0	0
Apple Juice—frozen	6 fl oz	90	20	0	0
Grape Juice	6 fl oz	120	10	0	0
Natural Grape Juice	6 fl oz	100	10	0	0
Natural Grape Juice—frozen	6 fl oz	115	20	0	0
Natural Style Apple Juice—frozen	6 fl oz	90	10	0	0
Sunglo					
100% Apple Juice	8.45 fl oz	130	65	0	0
100% Fruit Punch	8.45 fl oz	110	60	0	0
100% Grape Juice	8.45 fl oz	169	65	0	0
100% Grapefruit Juice	8.45 fl oz	94	75	0	0
Sunsweet					
Prune Juice	6 fl oz	130	20	0	0
Prune Juice w/Prune Pulp	6 fl oz	130	15	0	0
Tree Top					
Apple Cider	6 fl oz	90	10	0	0
Apple Juice from concentrate	6 fl oz	90	10	0	0
Apple Juice frozen concentrate	6 fl oz	90	10	0	0
Apple Pear Juice from concentrate	6 fl oz	90	10	0	0

Brand Name	Portion	Calories	Sodium (mg)	Fat (g)	Choles. (mg)
Apple Raspberry Juice from concentrate	6 fl oz	100	10	0	0
Unfiltered Apple Juice from concentrate	6 fl oz	90	10	0	0
Tropicana					
Orange Juice	6 fl oz	75	2	0	0
Orange Juice Premium	6 fl oz	75	2	0	0
Welch's					
Frozen Sweetened Grape Juice	6 fl oz	100	0	0	0
Grape Juice	6 fl oz	120	5	0	0
Sparkling Red Grape Juice	6 fl oz	128	30	0	0
Sparkling White Grape Juice	6 fl oz	120	30	0	0
100% White Grape Juice	6 fl oz	120	15	0	0
Welch's Orchard					
Frozen Grape Juice	6 fl oz	120	5	0	0
JUICE DRINKS					
Betty Crocker					
Squeezit Cherry	6.75 fl oz	110	5	0	0
Squeezit Grape	6.75 fl oz	110	5	0	0
Squeezit Orange	6.75 fl oz	110	5	0	0
Squeezit Red Punch	6.75 fl oz	110	5	0	0
Hawaiian Punch					
Fruit Juicy Red	6 fl oz	90	17	0	0
Punch Concentrate	6 fl oz	90	17	0	0
Juice Creations					
Nice & Natural Boysenberry Plus	6 fl oz	60	5	0	0
Nice & Natural Cherry Delight	6 fl oz	60	5	0	0
Nice & Natural Cranberry Delight	6 fl oz	68	4	0	0
Nice & Natural Papaya Delight	6 fl oz	80	5	0	0
Nice & Natural Piña Colada	6 fl oz	80	27	0	0
Nice & Natural Strawberry Delight	6 fl oz	60	5	0	0
Ocean Spray					
Cranapple Drink	6 fl oz	130	10	0	0
Cranberry Juice Cocktail	6 fl oz	110	10	0	0
Cranberry-Blueberry Drink	6 fl oz	120	5	0	0
Cranberry-Raspberry Drink	6 fl oz	110	10	0	0
Cranicot Drink	6 fl oz	110	15	0	0
Crantastic-Blended Juice Drink	6 fl oz	110	15	0	0
CranApple Drink	6 fl oz	130	10	0	0
CranGrape Drink	6 fl oz	130	5	0	0

Brand Name	Portion	Calories	Sodium (mg)	Fat (g)	Choles. (mg)
Ocean Spray cont.					
Low Calorie Cranberry Juice Cocktail	6 fl oz	40	10	0	0
Low Calorie CranApple Drink	6 fl oz	40	10	0	0
Low Calorie CranRaspberry Drink	6 fl oz	40	10	0	0
Mauna Lai Guava Fruit Drink	6 fl oz	100	10	0	0
Mauna Lai Guava-Passion Fruit Drink	6 fl oz	100	10	0	0
Pink Grapefruit Juice Cocktail	6 fl oz	80	15	0	0
Seneca					
Cranberry Juice Cocktail	6 fl oz	110	10	0	0
Sunny Delight					
Florida Citrus Punch	6 fl oz	90	55	0	0
Welch's					
Frozen CranApple Juice Drink	6 fl oz	120	0	0	0
Frozen CranRaspberry Drink	6 fl oz	110	0	0	0
Frozen Cranberry Juice Drink	6 fl oz	100	0	0	0
Welch's Orchard					
Cherry Fruit Juice Cocktail	6 fl oz	110	10	0	0
Frozen Cherry Fruit Juice Cocktail	6 fl oz	90	10	0	0
Wyler's					
Fruit Slush Fruit Punch	4 fl oz	180	15	1	0
Fruit Slush Grape	4 fl oz	180	15	1	0
Fruit Slush Orange	4 fl oz	180	15	1	0
POWDERED DRINKS					
Alpine					
Low Calorie Spiced Cider Mix	8 fl oz	16	30	0	0
Spiced Cider Mix	8 fl oz	80	20	0	0
Cragmont					
Lemonade Drink Mix	8 fl oz	90	15	0	0
Presweetened Mix Cherry	8 fl oz	90	15	0	0
Presweetened Mix Fruit Punch	8 fl oz	90	15	0	0
Presweetened Mix Grape	8 fl oz	90	15	0	0
Presweetened Mix Lemonade	8 fl oz	90	15	0	0
Presweetened Mix Orange	8 fl oz	90	15	0	0
Presweetened Mix Strawberry	8 fl oz	90	15	0	0
Punch Drink Mix	8 fl oz	90	15	0	0
Lucerne					
Coffee Instant Breakfast	1 envelope	130	140	0	0
Sugar Free Cocoa Mix	1 envelope	50	155	1	0

Brand Name	Portion	Calories	Sodium (mg)	Fat (g)	Choles. (mg)
Vanilla Instant Breakfast	1 envelope	130	160	0	0
Tang					
Orange Drink	6 fl oz	87	1	0	0
Orange Drink with Nutrasweet	6 fl oz	4	1	0	0
Town House					
Instant Orange Breakfast Drink	6 fl oz	90	0	0	0
Wyler					
Unsweetened Blackcherry	8 fl oz	2	20	0	0
Unsweetened Cherry	8 fl oz	2	20	0	0
Unsweetened Grape	8 fl oz	2	15	0	0

BREADS AND ROLLS

Bagels

Brand Name	Portion	Calories	Sodium (mg)	Fat (g)	Choles. (mg)
Lender's					
Blueberry Bagels	1	190	250	1	0
Onion Bagels	1	160	290	1	0
Plain Bagels	1	150	320	1	0
Raisin 'n Honey Bagels	1	200	310	1	0
Sara Lee					
Plain Bagels	1	230	540	1	0

Breads

Brand Name	Portion	Calories	Sodium (mg)	Fat (g)	Choles. (mg)
Roman Light					
Honey Wheatberry Bread	1 oz	40	105	0	0
Seven Grain Bread	1 oz	40	105	0	0
Wheat Bread	1 oz	40	105	0	0
Rubschlager					
Cocktail Pumpernickel Bread	2 slices	60	125	1	0
Cocktail Rye Bread	1 slice	50	135	1	0
Danish Pumpernickel Bread	1 slice	70	140	1	0
European Style Whole Grain Bread	1 slice	80	130	2	0
German Style Komissbrot	1 slice	70	150	1	0
Jewish Deli Rye Bread	1 slice	70	150	1	0
Sandwich Malt Bread	1 slice	90	180	2	0
Sandwich Rye Bread	1 slice	90	240	2	0
Sandwich Wheat Bread	1 slice	90	175	2	0
Swedish Limpa Rye Bread	1 slice	90	175	2	0
Westphalian Pumpernickel Bread	1 slice	60	95	1	0
100% Stone Ground Wheat	1 slice	70	130	1	0
Wonder					
White Bread	1 slice	70	140	1	0

Brand Name	Portion	Calories	Sodium (mg)	Fat (g)	Choles. (mg)
Buns, rolls, and muffins					
Duncan Hines					
Bakery Muffins: Cinnamon Swirl	1/12 pkg	190	240	6	0
Bakery Muffins: Bran/Honey Nut	1/12 pkg	190	215	6	0
Bakery Muffins: Cranberry Orange	1/12 pkg	190	210	7	0
Bakery Muffins: Blueberry	1/12 pkg	180	245	5	0
Bran and Honey Muffin Mix	1/12 pkg	110	165	3	0
Wild Blueberry Muffin Mix	1/12 pkg	100	150	3	0
Sara Lee					
Apple Cinnamon Muffins	1 muffin	220	280	8	0
Corn Muffins	1 muffin	250	330	13	0
Hearty Fruit Raisin Bran Muffin	1 muffin	220	400	7	0
Thomas'					
Honey Wheat English Muffins	1 muffin	130	200	1	0
Raisin English Muffins	1 muffin	153	200	2	0
Regular English Muffins	1 muffin	130	210	1	0
Sourdough English Muffins	1 muffin	130	208	1	0
OTHER					
Aunt Jemima					
Original Pancake & Waffle Mix	1.23 oz	120	610	1	0
Goodman's					
Passover Matzo	1 piece	129	0	0	0
Ideal					
Fiber w/Sesame Seeds Flatbread	2 slices	40	135	0	0
Whole Grain No Salt Flatbread	2 slices	43	0	0	0
Loma Linda					
Biscuits	2 biscuits	110	85	1	0
Ragú					
Quick Pizza Crust Mix	1.6 oz	170	360	2	0
BUTTER, MARGARINE, AND SPREADS					
Butter and margarine					
Chiffon					
Soft Whipped Margarine	1 tbps	70	80	8	0
Imperial					
Diet Margarine	1 tbsp	50	140	6	0
Soft Margarine	1 tbsp	100	95	11	0
Lucerne					
Corn Oil Margarine	1 tbsp	100	120	11	0
Margarine	1 tbsp	100	120	11	0

Brand Name	Portion	Calories	Sodium (mg)	Fat (g)	Choles. (mg)
Mazola					
Corn Oil Margarine	1 tbsp	100	100	11	0
Parkay					
Margarine	1 tbsp	100	115	11	0
Soft Margarine	1 tbsp	100	115	11	0
Squeeze Margarine	1 tbsp	100	115	11	0
Weight Watchers					
Reduced Calorie Margarine—Tub	1 tbsp	50	110	6	0
Spreads					
Gregg's					
Gold-n-Soft Lite Spread	1 tbsp	70	130	7	0
Imperial					
Light Spread	1 tbsp	60	110	6	0
Promise					
Sunflower Oil Spread	1 tbsp	90	90	10	0
Sunflower Oil Spread-Stick	1 tbsp	90	110	10	0
Shedd's					
Country Crock Spread	1 tbsp	70	100	7	0
Shedd's Corn Oil Spread	1 tbsp	70	100	7	0
CAKES, PASTRIES, AND FROSTINGS					
Cakes and pastries					
Batter-Lite					
Chocolate Lite Cake and Frosting	1/9 pkg	100	43	2	0
White Lite Cake and Frosting	1/9 pkg	100	36	2	0
Betty Crocker					
White Angel Food Cake Mix	1/12 pkg	150	300	0	0
Duncan Hines					
Black Forest Mousse Tiara Dessert	1/12 pkg	200	250	7	0
Brownie Mix	1/24 box	120	100	3	0
Butter Recipe Golden Cake Mix	1/12 pkg	190	160	4	0
Cherries & Cream Tiara Desert	1/12 pkg	180	240	5	0
Chewy Recipe Brownie Family Pack	1/24 pkg	100	85	2	0
Chocolate Amaretto Mousse Tiara Dessert	1/12 pkg	210	210	10	0
Chocolate Mousse Tiara Dessert	1/12 pkg	210	215	10	0
Peanut Butter Brownie Mix	1/24 box	120	100	5	0
Regular Chewy Brownie	1/16 box	100	85	2	0
Traditional Angel Food Cake Mix	1/12 mix	140	130	0	0

Brand Name	Portion	Calories	Sodium (mg)	Fat (g)	Choles. (mg)
Duncan Hines cont.					
Traditional Dark Dutch Fudge Cake	1/12 pkg	190	360	5	0
Traditional Devil's Food Cake Mix	1/12 pkg	190	360	5	0
Traditional French Vanilla Cake Mix	1/12 pkg	190	270	4	0
Traditional Lemon Supreme Cake Mix	1/12 pkg	190	270	4	0
Traditional Marble Fudge Cake	1/12 pkg	190	270	4	0
Traditional Pineapple Cake Mix	1/12 pkg	190	270	4	0
Traditional Spice Cake Mix	1/12 pkg	190	270	4	0
Traditional Strawberry Cake Mix	1/12 pkg	190	270	4	0
Traditional Swiss Chocolate Mix	1/12 pkg	190	360	5	0
Traditional White Cake Mix	1/12 pkg	190	250	4	0
Traditional Yellow Cake Mix	1/12 pkg	190	270	4	0
Kellogg's					
Blueberry Pop Tart	1 pastry	210	220	5	0
Brown Sugar Cinnamon Pop Tart	1 pastry	210	200	7	0
Frosted Blueberry Pop Tart	1 pastry	200	220	5	0
Frosted Cherry Pop Tart	1 pastry	210	230	5	0
Frosted Chocolate Fudge Pop Tart	1 pastry	200	230	4	0
Frosted Cinnamon Pop Tart	1 pastry	210	200	7	0
Frosted Dutch Apple Pop Tart	1 pastry	210	210	6	0
Frosted Strawberry Pop Tart	1 pastry	200	210	5	0
Strawberry Pop Tart	1 pastry	200	220	4	0
Frostings					
Duncan Hines					
Chocolate Frosting	1/12 contr	160	90	7	0
Milk Chocolate	1/12 contr	160	85	7	0
CANDIES					
Baker's					
Big Chips Milk Chocolate	1/4 cup	199	0	12	0
German Sweet Chocolate	1 oz sq	143	0	9	0
Real Semi-Sweet Chocolate Chips	1/4 cup	199	0	12	0
Semi-Sweet Chocolate	1 oz sq	135	0	9	0
Unsweetened Baking Chocolate	1 oz sq	140	1	15	0
Kraft					
Marshmallows	1 piece	25	10	0	0
Miniature Funmallows	10 pieces	18	0	0	0
Miniature Marshmallows	10 pieces	18	0	0	0
Party Mints	1 mint	8	0	0	0
Peanut Brittle	1 oz	140	140	5	0

Brand Name	Portion	Calories	Sodium (mg)	Fat (g)	Choles. (mg)
CEREALS, HOT					
General Mills					
Apple Cinnamon Instant Total Oatmeal	1.25 oz	130	140	2	0
Cinnamon/Almond/Raisin Total Oatmeal	1.5 oz	150	120	4	0
Mixed Nut Total Instant Oatmeal	1.3 oz	140	125	4	0
Quick Total Oatmeal	1 oz	90	115	2	0
Regular Instant Total Oatmeal	1 oz	90	220	2	0
Malt-O-Meal					
Chocolate Hot Cereal	1 oz	100	0	0	0
Quick Hot Cereal	1 oz	100	0	0	0
Nabisco					
Cream of Rice	1 oz	100	0	0	0
Cream of Wheat	1 oz	100	0	0	0
Instant Cream of Wheat	1 oz	100	0	0	0
Quick Cream of Wheat	1 oz	100	130	0	0
Quaker					
Instant Oatmeal Apples/ Cinnamon	1.25 oz	120	130	1	0
Instant Oatmeal Maple/Brown Sugar	1.5 oz	150	320	2	0
Instant Oatmeal Raisin/Date/ Walnut	1.3 oz	140	220	4	0
Instant Oatmeal Regular	1 oz	90	270	2	0
Old Fashioned Oats	1 oz	100	0	2	0
Quick Oats	1 oz	100	0	2	0
CEREALS, READY TO EAT					
Featherweight					
Corn Flakes	1 oz	110	10	0	0
General Mills					
Big B Clusters Cereal	1 oz	100	160	3	0
Cheerios	1¼ cups	110	290	2	0
Cinnamon Toast Crunch	¾ cup	120	220	3	0
Corn Total	1 cup	110	280	1	0
Crispy Wheats 'n Raisins	¾ cup	110	180	1	0
Fiber One	½ cup	60	140	1	0
Golden Grahams	¾ cup	110	280	1	0
Honey Nut Cheerios	¾ cup	110	250	1	0
Kix	1½ cups	110	240	0	0
Oatmeal Raisin Crisp	½ cup	150	140	2	0
Total	1 cup	100	280	1	0

Brand Name	Portion	Calories	Sodium (mg)	Fat (g)	Choles. (mg)
General Mills cont.					
Trix	1 cup	110	170	1	0
Wheaties	1 cup	110	280	1	0
Health Valley					
Bran Cereal with Apples & Cinnamon	1 oz	109	10	1	0
Bran Cereal w/Raisins	1 oz	105	10	1	0
Real Cereal Almond Crunch	1 oz	119	5	3	0
Kashi					
Puffed 7 Whole Grain w/Sesame	¾ oz	74	2	1	0
Kellogg's					
All-Bran	⅓ cup	70	260	1	0
All-Bran w/Extra Fiber	½ cup	60	270	1	0
Apple Cinnamon Squares	½ cup	90	5	0	0
Apple Jacks	1 cup	110	125	0	0
Bran Flakes	⅔ cup	90	220	0	0
Cocoa Krispies	¾ cup	110	190	0	0
Corn Flakes	1 cup	100	290	0	0
Corn Pops	1 cup	110	90	0	0
Cracklin' Oat Bran	½ cup	110	140	4	0
Crispix	1 cup	110	220	0	0
Froot Loops	1 cup	110	125	1	0
Frosted Flakes	¾ cup	110	200	0	0
Frosted Mini-Wheats	4 biscuits	100	5	0	0
Honey Smacks	¾ cup	110	70	0	0
Just Right Fruit Nut & Flake	¾ cup	140	190	0	0
Mueslix Bran	½ cup	130	100	2	0
Mueslix Five Grain Cereal	½ cup	150	60	2	0
Nut & Honey Crunch	⅔ cup	110	200	1	0
Nutri-Grain Almond Raisin	⅔ cup	140	220	2	0
Nutri-Grain Biscuits	⅔ cup	90	0	0	0
Nutri-Grain Nuggets	¼ cup	90	110	0	0
Nutri-Grain Wheat	⅔ cup	100	170	0	0
Product 19	1 cup	100	320	0	0
Raisin Bran	¾ cup	120	220	1	0
Raisin Squares	½ cup	90	0	0	0
Rice Krispies	1 cup	110	290	0	0
Special K	1 cup	110	230	0	0
Strawberry Squares	½ cup	90	5	0	0
Post					
Alpha Bits	1 cup	111	180	1	0
Alpha Bits Unsweetened	1 cup	111	180	1	0

Brand Name	Portion	Calories	Sodium (mg)	Fat (g)	Choles. (mg)
Crispy Critters	½ cup	87	159	0	0
Crunchy Stars	1 cup	111	180	1	0
Fortified Oat Flakes	⅔ cup	106	243	1	0
Fruit & Fiber Cinnamon Apple Crisp	½ cup	92	179	1	0
Fruit & Fiber Dates/Raisins/ Walnuts	½ cup	89	179	1	0
Grape Nuts	¼ cup	105	190	1	0
Grape Nuts Flakes	⅞ cup	104	170	1	0
Honeycomb	1⅓ cup	111	159	0	0
Pebbles Fruity	⅞ cup	113	145	1	0
Raisin Bran	½ cup	87	159	0	0
Super Golden Crisp	⅞ cup	105	45	0	0
40% Bran Flakes	⅔ cup	106	243	1	0
Quaker					
Cap'n Crunch	¾ cup	120	240	2	0
Cap'n Crunch Crunchberries	¾ cup	120	250	2	0
Life	⅔ cup	100	190	2	0
Oat Squares	1 oz	100	160	2	0
Raisin-Date Natural Cereal	¼ cup	132	15	5	0
100% Natural Cereal	¼ cup	130	15	6	0
Ralston					
Corn Chex	1 cup	110	328	1	0
Rice Chex	1⅛ cups	110	252	1	0

COFFEE CREAMERS

Brand Name	Portion	Calories	Sodium (mg)	Fat (g)	Choles. (mg)
Cremora					
Non-dairy Creamer	1 tsp	—	5	1	0
Lucerne					
Non-dairy Creamer	½ oz	26	5	2	0
Rich's					
Coffee Rich Non-dairy Creamer	½ oz	30	11	2	0

COOKIES

Brand Name	Portion	Calories	Sodium (mg)	Fat (g)	Choles. (mg)
Duncan Hines					
Golden Sugar Cookie Mix	2 cookies	130	65	6	0
Oatmeal Raisin Cookies	2 cookies	110	75	5	0
Oatmeal Raisin Cookie Mix	2 cookies	130	65	6	0
Peanut Butter Cookie Mix	2 cookies	140	115	7	0
Health Valley					
Apple Bakes Fruit Bars	2 bars	164	35	4	0
Date Pecan Fancy Fruit Cookie	2 cookies	70	45	2	0

Brand Name	Portion	Calories	Sodium (mg)	Fat (g)	Choles. (mg)
Health Valley cont.					
Peanut Butter Cookies	2 cookies	70	55	2	0
Raisin Bakes Fruit Bars	2 bars	160	35	4	0
Sunshine					
Golden Fruit Cookie	2 cookies	150	80	3	0
Grahamy Bears	9 cookies	130	160	5	0
Sugar Wafers	3 wafers	130	40	6	0
Vienna Fingers	2 cookies	140	125	6	0
CRACKERS					
Chico-San					
Rice Cake Sesame, Salted	1 cake	35	10	0	0
Rice Cake Sesame, Unsalted	1 cake	35	0	0	0
Finn Crisp					
Dark Crisp Bread Caraway Seeds	2 crisps	38	130	0	0
Health Valley					
Amaranth Graham Crackers	7 crackers	139	110	3	0
Oat Bran Graham Cracker	7 crackers	119	85	3	0
Quaker					
Corn Grain Cakes	1 cake	35	55	0	0
Multi Grain Rice Cakes	1 cake	35	30	0	0
Rye Grain Cakes	1 cake	35	50	0	0
Sesame Rice Cakes	1 cake	35	36	0	0
Unsalted Sesame Rice Cakes	1 cake	35	0	0	0
Wheat Grain Cakes	1 cake	35	50	0	0
Sunshine					
Animal Crackers	14 crackers	120	180	3	0
Cheez-Its	12 crackers	70	135	4	0
Cheez-Its Low Salt	12 crackers	70	65	4	0
Graham Crackers	1 cracker	60	90	2	0
Hi Ho Crackers	4 crackers	80	125	5	0
Krispy Saltines	5 crackers	60	210	1	0
Krispy Unsalted Tops	5 crackers	60	120	1	0
Wheat Wafers	8 wafers	80	190	4	0
Wasa					
Breakfast Crispbread	1 slice	50	65	1	0
Extra Crisp Crackerbread	1 slice	25	40	1	0
Extra-Thin Flatbread	3 slices	48	119	0	0
Fiber Plus Crispbread	1 slice	35	65	1	0
Golden Rye Crispbread	1 slice	35	55	0	0
Hearty Rye Crispbread	1 slice	45	70	0	0
Savory Sesame Crispbread	1 slice	30	40	1	0

Brand Name	Portion	Calories	Sodium (mg)	Fat (g)	Choles. (mg)
DESSERTS AND TOPPINGS					
Frozen desserts					
Dole					
Fruit Sorbet Peach	4 fl oz	120	11	0	0
Fruit Sorbet Pineapple	4 fl oz	120	10	0	0
Fruit Sorbet Raspberry	4 fl oz	110	9	0	0
Fruit Sorbet Strawberry	4 fl oz	110	11	0	0
Piña Colada Fruit 'n Juice	2.5 fl oz	90	2	3	0
Gelatins					
Jell-Well					
Cherry Gelatin	½ cup	80	70	0	0
Lemon Gelatin	½ cup	80	70	0	0
Lime Gelatin	½ cup	80	70	0	0
Mixed Fruit Gelatin	½ cup	80	70	0	0
Orange Gelatin	½ cup	80	70	0	0
Raspberry Gelatin	½ cup	80	70	0	0
Strawberry Gelatin	½ cup	80	70	0	0
Strawberry/Banana Gelatin	½ cup	80	70	0	0
Sugar Free Orange	½ cup	8	50	0	0
Sugar Free Raspberry	½ cup	8	50	0	0
Sugar Free Strawberry	½ cup	8	50	0	0
Sugar Free Strawberry Banana	½ cup	8	50	0	0
Jell-O					
Cherry Gelatin	½ cup	80	70	0	0
Lemon Gelatin	½ cup	80	73	0	0
Lime Gelatin	½ cup	80	56	0	0
Orange Gelatin	½ cup	80	50	0	0
Raspberry Gelatin	½ cup	80	50	0	0
Strawberry Banana Gelatin	½ cup	80	50	0	0
Strawberry Gelatin	½ cup	80	50	0	0
Sugar Free Cherry Gelatin	½ cup	8	79	0	0
Sugar Free Hawaiian Pineapple Gelatin	½ cup	8	49	0	
Sugar Free Lemon Gelatin	½ cup	8	49	0	0
Sugar Free Lime Gelatin	½ cup	8	59	0	0
Sugar Free Mixed Fruit Gelatin	½ cup	8	48	0	0
Sugar Free Raspberry Gelatin	½ cup	8	51	0	0
Sugar Free Strawberry Banana Gelatin	½ cup	8	63	0	0
Sugar Free Strawberry Gelatin	½ cup	8	63	0	0
Sugar Free Triple Berry Gelatin	½ cup	8	49	0	0
Wild Strawberry Gelatin	½ cup	80	73	0	0

Brand Name	Portion	Calories	Sodium (mg)	Fat (g)	Choles. (mg)
Puddings					
General Foods					
Minute Tapioca	1 tbsp	31	0	0	0
Toppings					
Baker's					
Dream Whip Topping	¼ cup	199	0	12	0
Cool Whip					
Extra Creamy Topping	1 tbsp	15	3	1	0
Non-dairy Topping	1 tbsp	11	1	1	0
D-Zerta					
Whipped Topping w/Nutrasweet	1 tbsp	160	6	0	0
Kraft					
Marshmallow Creme	1 oz	90	15	0	0
DRESSING AND SPREADS					
Salad dressings					
Catalina					
Reduced Calorie Dressing	1 tbsp	16	125	0	0
Good Seasons					
Low Calorie Italian Dressing	1 tbsp	6	31	0	0
Herb Magic					
Italian Salad Dressing	1 tbsp	4	129	0	0
Vinaigrette Salad Dressing	1 tbsp	6	167	0	0
Kraft					
Creamy Italian Dressing	1 tbsp	60	120	6	0
Oil-Free Italian Dressing	1 tbsp	4	210	0	0
Reduced Calorie Bacon & Tomato	1 tbsp	30	150	2	0
Reduced Calorie Chunky Blue Cheese	1 tbsp	30	240	2	0
Reduced Calorie Creamy Buttermilk	1 tbsp	30	125	3	0
Reduced Calorie Creamy Cucumber	1 tbsp	30	230	3	0
Reduced Calorie Creamy Italian	1 tbsp	25	125	2	0
Richelieu					
Reduced Calorie Western Dressing	1 tbsp	35	125	1	0
Western Dressing	1 tbsp	70	105	5	0

Brand Name	Portion	Calories	Sodium (mg)	Fat (g)	Choles. (mg)
Seven Seas					
Buttermilk Recipe	1 tbsp	80	130	8	0
Red Wine Vinegar & Oil	1 tbsp	60	265	7	0
Viva Italian Dressing	1 tbsp	70	320	7	0
Wish-Bone					
Chunky Blue Cheese Dressing	1 tbsp	70	150	8	0
Deluxe French Dressing	1 tbsp	60	80	6	0
Italian Dressing	1 tbsp	45	280	4	0
Lite Class Dijon Vinaigrette	1 tbsp	25	190	2	0
Lite Italian Dressing	1 tbsp	6	210	1	0
Lite Onion 'n Chive Dressing	1 tbsp	35	160	3	0
Lite Russian Dressing	1 tbsp	25	140	1	0
Ranch Dressing	1 tbsp	80	150	8	0
Russian Dressing	1 tbsp	45	150	3	0
Sweet 'n Spicy French Dressing	1 tbsp	70	150	6	0

EGG SUBSTITUTES

Brand Name	Portion	Calories	Sodium (mg)	Fat (g)	Choles. (mg)
Fleischmann's					
Egg Beaters	¼ cup	25	80	0	0
Morningstar Farm					
Scramblers Cholesterol Free Egg Product	¼ cup	60	130	3	0

ENTRÉES

Brand Name	Portion	Calories	Sodium (mg)	Fat (g)	Choles. (mg)
Health Valley					
Mild Vegetarian Chili/No Salt	4 oz	146	25	6	0
Spicy Vegetarian Chili/No Salt	4 oz	146	25	6	0
Hunt's					
Manwich Extra Thick & Chunky	2.5 oz	40	470	0	0

FLOURS, GRAINS, AND LEGUMES

Flours

Brand Name	Portion	Calories	Sodium (mg)	Fat (g)	Choles. (mg)
Fisher					
Rye Flour	1 cup	450	0	2	0
General Mills					
Softsilk Flour	4 oz	100	0	0	0
Gold Medal					
All Purpose Flour	4 oz	400	0	1	0
High Protein Flour for Bread	4 oz	400	0	1	0
Unbleached Flour	4 oz	400	0	1	0
Whole Wheat Blend	4 oz	370	0	2	0
Whole Wheat Flour	4 oz	390	0	2	0

Brand Name	Portion	Calories	Sodium (mg)	Fat (g)	Choles. (mg)
Flours *cont.*					
Goodman's					
Passover Matzo Meal	1 cup	514	5	1	0
La Pina					
Flour	4 oz	400	0	1	0
Mrs. Wright					
All Purpose Flour	1 cup	400	0	1	0
Ovenjoy					
Flour	1 cup	400	0	1	0
Grains					
Heinz					
Couscous	1¾ oz	180	5	0	0
Tabouleh	1⅙ oz	120	230	1	0
Kretchmer					
Wheat Germ	1 oz	100	0	3	0
Mrs. Wright's					
White Corn Meal Self Rising	1 oz	100	0	0	0
Yellow Corn Meal	1 oz	100	0	0	0
Van Camp's					
Golden Hominy	1 cup	128	701	1	0
White Hominy	1 cup	138	708	1	0
Legumes					
Hurst					
Hambeens 15 Bean Soup	1 cup	220	130	1	0
Van Camp's					
Dark Red Kidney Beans	1 cup	182	732	1	0
New Orleans Style Kidney Beans	1 cup	178	793	1	0
FRUITS, CANNED					
Del Monte					
Bartlett Pear Halves	½ cup	80	10	0	0
Crushed Pineapple in Juice	½ cup	70	10	0	0
Freestone Peach Slices	½ cup	90	10	0	0
Fruit Cocktail	½ cup	80	10	0	0
Lite Fruit Cocktail	½ cup	50	10	0	0
Lite Sliced Peaches	½ cup	50	10	0	0
Mixed Fruit Cup	5 oz	100	10	0	0
Pineapple Tidbits in Juice	½ cup	70	10	0	0
Sliced Pineapple in Juice	½ cup	90	10	0	0
Yellow Cling Peach Halves	½ cup	80	10	0	0
Yellow Cling Peach Slices	½ cup	80	10	0	0

Brand Name	Portion	Calories	Sodium (mg)	Fat (g)	Choles. (mg)
Dole					
Chuck Pineapple in Heavy Syrup	½ cup	90	10	0	0
Chunk Pineapple in Juice	½ cup	70	10	1	0
Crushed Pineapple in Heavy Syrup	½ cup	90	10	0	0
Crushed Pineapple in Juice	½ cup	70	10	0	0
Mandarin Oranges	½ cup	70	8	0	0
Pineapple Tidbits in Juice	½ cup	70	10	0	0
Sliced Pineapple in Heavy Syrup	2 slices	90	10	0	0
Sliced Pineapple in Juice	2 slices	70	10	0	0
Mott's					
Apple Sauce Regular	4 oz	88	0	0	0
Chunky Apple Sauce	4 oz	57	7	0	0
Cinnamon Apple Sauce	4 oz	72	0	0	0
Natural Apple Sauce	4 oz	44	0	0	0
Regular Apple Sauce	4 oz	88	0	0	0
Ocean Spray					
CranOrange Sauce	2 oz	100	15	0	0
CranRaspberry Sauce	2 oz	90	15	0	0
Jellied Cranberry Sauce	2 oz	90	15	0	0
Whole Berry Cranberry Sauce	2 oz	90	15	0	0
Seneca					
Applesauce	½ cup	90	20	0	0
100% Natural Applesauce	½ cup	50	20	0	0
Sunsweet					
Ready to Serve Prunes	½ cup	120	10	0	0
Tree Top					
Cinnamon Applesauce	½ cup	80	0	0	0
Natural Applesauce	½ cup	60	0	0	0
Original Applesauce	½ cup	90	10	0	0
DRIED FRUITS					
Dromedary					
Dates, Chopped	¼ cup	130	0	0	0
Mariani					
Dried Apricots	¼ cup	140	10	0	0
Dried Pears	¼ cup	150	10	0	0
Pitted Prunes	¼ cup	140	10	1	0
Nabisco					
Dates, Pitted	5 dates	100	0	0	0

Brand Name	Portion	Calories	Sodium (mg)	Fat (g)	Choles. (mg)
Dried Fruits *cont.*					
Sun Giant					
Chopped Dates	1 cup	490	1	1	0
Pitted Dates	10 dates	220	1	1	0
Raisins	2.8 oz	260	25	0	0
Sun-Maid					
Apple Chunks	2 oz	150	40	0	0
Apricots	2 oz	140	10	0	0
Calimyrna Figs	½ cup	250	10	2	0
Fruit Bits	2 oz	160	40	0	0
Golden Raisins	½ cup	260	10	0	0
Mission Figs	½ cup	210	20	1	0
Mixed Fruit	2 oz	150	20	0	0
Muscat Raisins	½ cup	270	25	1	0
Peaches	2 oz	140	10	0	0
Seedless Raisins	1 oz	96	5	0	0
Zante Currants	½ cup	210	15	0	0
Sunsweet					
Bite-sized Pitted Prunes	2 oz	120	10	0	0
Extra Large Prunes	2 oz	120	10	0	0
Large Prunes	2 oz	120	10	0	0
Medium Prunes	2 oz	120	10	0	0
Pitted Prunes	2 oz	120	10	0	0
INGREDIENT FOODS					
Baker's					
Angel Flake Coconut—Bag	⅓ cup	118	73	8	0
Angel Flake Coconut—Can	⅓ cup	113	5	9	0
Big Chips Semi Sweet	¼ cup	199	0	12	0
Premium Shred Coconut	⅓ cup	138	84	10	0
Calumet					
Baking Powder	1 tbsp	2	408	0	0
Kingsford's					
Corn Starch	1 tbsp	30	0	0	0
Sure-Jell					
Fruit Pectin	¼ pkg	38	1	0	0
JAMS, JELLIES, AND SPREADS					
Country Pure					
Apricot Jam	2 tsp	35	10	0	0
Blackberry Jam	2 tsp	35	10	0	0
Red Cherry Jam	2 tsp	35	10	0	0

Brand Name	Portion	Calories	Sodium (mg)	Fat (g)	Choles. (mg)
Red Raspberry Jam	2 tsp	35	10	0	0
Strawberry Jam	2 tsp	35	10	0	0
Empress					
Apple Jelly	2 tsp	35	10	0	0
Apricot Pineapple Preserves	2 tsp	35	10	0	0
Apricot Preserves	2 tsp	35	10	0	0
Black Cherry Preserves	2 tsp	35	10	0	0
Black Raspberry Preserves	2 tsp	35	10	0	0
Blackberry Jelly	2 tsp	35	10	0	0
Boysenberry Preserves	2 tsp	35	10	0	0
Calif. Orange Marmalade	2 tsp	35	10	0	0
Concord Grape Jam	2 tsp	35	10	0	0
Grape Jam	2 tsp	35	10	0	0
Mixed Fruit Jelly	2 tsp	35	10	0	0
Peach Pineapple Preserves	2 tsp	35	10	0	0
Peach Preserves	2 tsp	35	10	0	0
Plum Preserves	2 tsp	35	10	0	0
Red Cherry Preserves	2 tsp	35	10	0	0
Red Currant Jelly	2 tsp	35	10	0	0
Red Raspberry Preserves	2 tsp	35	10	0	0
Seedless Blackberry Preserves	2 tsp	35	10	0	0
Spiced Apple Butter	2 tsp	35	10	0	0
Strawberry Preserves	2 tsp	35	10	0	0
King Kelly					
Orange Marmalade	1 tsp	18	0	0	0
Mary Ellen					
Apricot Jam	2 tsp	35	0	0	0
Grape Jam	2 tsp	35	0	0	0
Grape Jelly	2 tsp	35	0	0	0
Red Raspberry Jam	2 tsp	35	0	0	0
Seedless Blackberry Jam	2 tsp	35	0	0	0
Strawberry Jam	2 tsp	35	0	0	0
Strawberry Jelly	2 tsp	35	0	0	0
Piedmont					
Grape Jam	2 tsp	36	10	0	0
Grape Jelly	2 tsp	36	10	0	0
Red Raspberry Preserves	2 tsp	36	10	0	0
Strawberry Preserves	2 tsp	36	10	0	0
Smucker's					
Apricot Preserves	2 tsp	35	10	0	0

Brand Name	Portion	Calories	Sodium (mg)	Fat (g)	Choles. (mg)
Smucker's cont.					
Apricot-Pineapple Preserves	2 tsp	35	0	0	0
Boysenberry Preserves	2 tsp	35	0	0	0
Grape Jam	2 tsp	35	0	0	0
Grape Jelly	2 tsp	35	0	0	0
Low Sugar Boysenberry Spread	2 tsp	16	0	0	0
Low Sugar Grape Spread	2 tsp	16	0	0	0
Low Sugar Orange Marmalade	2 tsp	16	0	0	0
Low Sugar Red Raspberry Spread	2 tsp	16	0	0	0
Low Sugar Strawberry Spread	2 tsp	16	0	0	0
Mint Apple Jelly	2 tsp	35	0	0	0
Orange Marmalade	2 tsp	35	0	0	0
Red Plum Jam	2 tsp	35	0	0	0
Red Raspberry Jam	2 tsp	35	0	0	0
Red Raspberry Preserves	2 tsp	35	0	0	0
Seedless Black Raspberry Jam	2 tsp	35	0	0	0
Seedless Blackberry Jam	2 tsp	35	0	0	0
Seedless Boysenberry Jam	2 tsp	35	0	0	0
Seedless Red Raspberry Jam	2 tsp	35	0	0	0
Seedless Strawberry Jam	2 tsp	35	0	0	0
Spiced Apple Butter	2 tsp	25	0	0	0
Strawberry Jam	2 tsp	35	0	0	0
Strawberry Preserves	2 tsp	35	0	0	0
Welch's					
Concord Grape Jam	2 tsp	35	5	0	0
Concord Grape Jelly	2 tsp	35	5	0	0
Squeezable Grape Jelly	2 tsp	35	5	0	0
Squeezable Strawberry Preserves	2 tsp	35	5	0	0

MEATS AND SEAFOODS

Brand Name	Portion	Calories	Sodium (mg)	Fat (g)	Choles. (mg)
Morningstar Farm					
Cholesterol Free Breakfast Patties	2 patties	190	870	11	0
Cholesterol Free Breakfast Strips	3 strips	80	330	6	0
Cholesterol Free Breakfast Links	3 links	180	480	12	0
Grillers Cholesterol Free Patties	1 pattie	180	320	12	0

NUTS AND NUT BUTTERS
Nuts

Brand Name	Portion	Calories	Sodium (mg)	Fat (g)	Choles. (mg)
Azar					
Almond Slices	1 oz	170	0	15	0
Black Walnuts	1 oz	170	0	16	0
Blanched Slivered Almonds	1 oz	170	0	15	0
Natural Whole Almonds	1 oz	170	0	15	0

Brand Name	Portion	Calories	Sodium (mg)	Fat (g)	Choles. (mg)
Pecan Chips	1 oz	210	0	21	0
Pecan Halves	1 oz	210	0	21	0
Pecan Pieces	1 oz	210	0	21	0
Pecan Slices	1 oz	210	0	21	0
Walnut Chips	1 oz	190	0	19	0
Walnut Halves	1 oz	190	0	19	0
Blue Diamond					
Dry Roasted Unsalted Almonds	1 oz	179	5	14	0
Roasted Salted Almonds	1 oz	150	110	15	0
Smokehouse Almonds	1 oz	150	115	14	0
Diamond					
Chopped Walnuts	1 oz	190	5	19	0
Shelled Walnuts	1 oz	190	5	19	0
Eagle Snacks					
Honey Roast Cashews	1 oz	170	170	12	0
Honey Roast Peanut/Cashew Mix	1 oz	170	170	13	0
Honey Roast Peanuts	1 oz	170	170	13	0
Planters					
Mixed Nuts	1 oz	180	130	16	0
Oil Roasted Cashew Halves	1 oz	170	135	14	0
Roasted Unsalted Mixed Nuts	1 oz	170	0	15	0
Sweet & Crunchy Peanuts	1 oz	140	20	8	0
Unsalted Dry Roasted Peanuts	1 oz	170	0	15	0
Nut butters					
Country Pure					
Chunky Peanut Butter	2 tbsp	190	130	16	0
Creamy Peanut Butter	2 tbsp	190	150	16	0
Health Valley					
Unsalted Chunky Peanut Butter	1 tbsp	91	1	7	0
Unsalted Ceamy Peanut Butter	1 tbsp	83	1	7	0
Jif					
Creamy Peanut Butter	2 tbsp	190	155	16	0
Extra Crunchy Peanut Butter	2 tbsp	190	130	16	0
Nu Made					
Chunky Peanut Butter	2 tbsp	190	130	16	0
Creamy Peanut Butter	2 tbsp	190	150	16	0
Real Roast					
Chunky Peanut Butter	2 tbsp	190	130	16	0

Brand Name	Portion	Calories	Sodium (mg)	Fat (g)	Choles. (mg)
Nut butters *cont.*					
Skippy					
Creamy Peanut Butter	2 tbsp	190	150	17	0
Super Chunk Peanut Butter	2 tbsp	190	130	17	0
OILS AND SHORTENINGS					
Crisco					
Butter Flavor Shortening	1 tbsp	110	0	12	0
Corn Oil	1 tbsp	120	0	14	0
Oil	1 tbsp	120	0	14	0
Shortening	1 tbsp	110	0	12	0
Vegetable Oil	1 tbsp	120	0	14	0
Hollywood					
Peanut Oil	1 tbsp	120	0	14	0
Safflower Oil	1 tbsp	120	0	14	0
Sunflower Oil	1 tbsp	120	0	14	0
Mazola					
Corn Oil	1 tbsp	120	0	14	0
Nu Made					
Shortening	1 tbsp	110	0	12	0
Vegetable Oil	1 tbsp	120	0	14	0
Orville Redenbacher's					
Buttery Flavor Popping Oil	1 tbsp	120	0	14	0
Pam					
Butter Flavor Cooking Spray	0.8 gm	7	0	1	0
Vegetable Cooking Spray	0.8 gm	7	0	1	0
Planters					
Peanut Oil	1 tbsp	130	0	14	0
Puritan					
100% Pure Vegetable Oil	1 tbsp	120	0	14	0
Weight Watchers					
Buttery Spray	1 second	2	0	1	0
Cooking Spray	1 second	2	0	1	0
Wesson					
Corn Oil	1 tbsp	120	0	14	0
Sunflower Oil	1 tbsp	120	0	14	0
Vegetable Oil	1 tbsp	120	0	14	0
PASTA					
American Beauty					
Coiled Vermicelli	2 oz	210	0	1	0
Curly Roni	2 oz	210	0	1	0
Elbo Roni	2 oz	210	0	1	0

Brand Name	Portion	Calories	Sodium (mg)	Fat (g)	Choles. (mg)
Fettucine	2 oz	220	10	3	0
Lasagne	2 oz	210	0	1	0
Long Spaghetti	2 oz	210	0	1	0
Mostaccioli	2 oz	210	0	1	0
Rainbow Shells	2 oz	210	30	1	0
Rainbow Twirls	2 oz	210	30	1	0
Roni Mac	2 oz	210	30	1	0
Rotini	2 oz	210	0	1	0
Salad Mac	2 oz	210	0	1	0
Shell Roni	2 oz	210	0	1	0
Spaghetti	2 oz	210	0	1	0
Thin Spaghetti	2 oz	210	0	1	0
Vermicelli	2 oz	210	0	1	0
Creamette					
Elbow Macaroni	2 oz	210	15	1	0
Fettucine	2 oz	210	20	1	0
Lasagna	2 oz	210	20	1	0
Linguini	2 oz	210	15	1	0
Mostaccioli	2 oz.	210	15	1	0
Rainbow Rotini	2 oz.	210	5	1	0
Rigatoni	2 oz	210	15	1	0
Rotini	2 oz.	210	15	1	0
Spaghetti	2 oz	210	15	1	0
Thin Spaghetti	2 oz	210	15	1	0
Vermicelli	2 ozz	210	15	1	0
RICE					
Birds Eye					
Int'l French Style	½ cup	117	635	1	0
Long Grain/Wild Rice-a-Roni	1.3 oz	130	780	1	0
Heinz					
Beef Flavored Rice	1 oz	100	390	0	0
Chicken Flavored Rice	1 oz	100	240	1	0
Long/Wild Rice	½ cup	100	440	1	0
Rice Pilaf	1 oz	100	370	0	0
Spanish Rice Pilaf	1 oz	100	360	0	0
Kashhi					
Whole Grain & Sesame Pilaf	2 oz dry	177	5	1	0
Konriko					
Wild Pecan Rice	½ cup	89	0	1	0
Scotch Buy					
Long Grain Rice	⅓ cup	110	0	0	0

Brand Name	Portion	Calories	Sodium (mg)	Fat (g)	Choles. (mg)
Rice *cont.*					
Town House					
Long Grain White Rice	⅙ cup	110	0	0	0
Medium Grain Rice	⅙ cup	110	0	0	0
SAUCES/GRAVIES AND CONDIMENTS					
Sauces/gravies					
Hunt's					
Italian Tomato Sauce	4 oz	30	670	0	0
No Salt Tomato Sauce	4 oz	30	25	0	0
Tomato Sauce	4 oz	30	670	0	0
Tomato Sauce w/Garlic	4 oz	30	670	0	0
Kikkoman					
Lite Soy Sauce	½ tsp	2	100	0	0
Milder Soy Sauce	½ tsp	—	85	0	0
Soy Sauce	½ tsp	3	160	0	0
Stir-Fry Sauce	½ tsp	3	60	0	0
Sukiyaki Sauce	½ tsp	—	75	0	0
Sweet & Sour Sauce	1 tbsp	18	63	0	0
Teriyaki Baste & Glaze	1 tsp	9	140	0	0
Teriyaki Sauce	½ tsp	3	105	0	0
Tonkatsu Sauce	½ tsp	—	50	0	0
Kingsford					
Masterpiece Mesquite BBQ Sauce	1 tbsp	30	250	0	0
Masterpiece Original BBQ Sauce	1 tbsp	30	250	0	0
Kraft					
BBQ Sauce	2 tbsp	40	510	1	0
Hickory Smoked BBQ Sauce	2 tbsp	40	510	1	0
Mesquite Smoked BBQ Sauce	2 tbsp	45	420	1	0
Thick N Spicy BBQ Sauce	2 tbsp	50	510	1	0
Thick N Spicy Hickory Smoked BBQ Sauce	2 tbsp	50	510	1	0
Thick N Spicy Kansas City BBQ Sauce	2 tbsp	60	320	1	0
Old El Paso					
Hot Picante Sauce	2 tbsp	8	310	0	0
Medium Picante Sauce	2 tbsp	8	310	0	0
Mild Picante Sauce	2 tbsp	8	330	0	0
Ragú					
Chunky Gardenstyle Spaghetti Sauce	4 oz	80	400	2	0

Brand Name	Portion	Calories	Sodium (mg)	Fat (g)	Choles. (mg)
Chunky Spaghetti Sauce Green Pepper/Mushroom	4 oz	80	400	2	0
Chunky Spaghetti Sauce Mushroom/Onion	4 oz	80	400	2	0
Garden Chunky Italian Combination	4 oz	80	400	2	0
Homestyle Spaghetti Sauce	4 oz	70	400	2	0
Homestyle Spaghetti Sauce Mushroom	4 oz	70	400	2	0
Quick Pizza Sauce—Pepperoni	1.7 oz	50	330	2	0
Quick Pizza Sauce—Traditional	1.7 oz	40	300	2	0
Thick & Hearty Spaghetti Sauce	4 oz	140	530	2	0
Thick & Hearty Spaghetti Sauce —Meat	4 oz	140	530	2	0
Thick & Hearty Spaghetti Sauce —Mushroom	4 oz	140	530	2	0
Traditional Spaghetti Sauce w/ Extra Garlic	4 oz	70	400	2	0
Town House					
Chunk Style Spaghetti Sauce	4 oz	80	400	2	0
Tomato Sauce	8 oz	80	1,360	0	0
Condiments					
Del Monte					
Tomato Catsup	¼ cup	60	675	0	0
General Mills					
Bac-Os	2 tsp	25	90	1	0
SEASONINGS					
Adolph's					
Natural Unsalted Tenderizer/ Unseasoned	1 tsp	—	10	0	0
Natural Unsalted Tenderizer w/Spices	1 tsp	—	10	0	0
Morton					
Iodized Table Salt	1 tsp	0	2,300	0	0
Kosher Salt	1 tsp	0	1,880	0	0
Lite Salt Mixture	½ tsp	0	550	0	0
Plain Table Salt	1 tsp	0	2,300	0	0
Salt Substitute	1 tsp	0	1	0	0
Mrs. Dash					
Extra Spicy Seasoning	1 tsp	—	5	1	0
Salt Free Seasoning	1 tsp	—	3	0	0

Brand Name	Portion	Calories	Sodium (mg)	Fat (g)	Choles. (mg)
Mrs. Dash cont.					
Salt Free Seasoning–Low Pepper					
No Garlic	1 tsp	—	4	1	0
Seasoning Lemon/Herb	1 tsp	—	4	1	0
Parsley Patch					
All-Purpose Blend—Salt Free	1 tsp	0	0	0	0
Oriental Blend Salt Free	1 tsp	0	0	0	0
Shake 'N Bake					
Original BBQ Recipe/Chicken	¼ pouch	92	837	2	0
Original BBQ Recipe/Pork	¼ pouch	81	601	1	0
Season Salt Substitute	1 tsp	0	0	0	0
The HVR Company					
Kitchen Bouquet	½ tsp	6	10	0	0

SNACKS

Brand Name	Portion	Calories	Sodium (mg)	Fat (g)	Choles. (mg)
Doritos					
Nacho Cheese Tortilla Chips	1 oz	140	250	7	0
Taco Flavor Chips	1 oz	140	230	6	0
Tortilla Chips Regular	1 oz	140	230	6	0
Eagle Snacks					
Cantina Tortilla Nachos	1 oz	150	190	8	0
Cantina Tortilla Chips Regular	1 oz	150	140	8	0
Cheese Crunch	1 oz	160	300	10	0
Eagle Pretzels	1 oz	110	570	2	0
Extra Crunchy BBQ Chips	1 oz	150	220	8	0
Extra Crunchy Chips	1 oz	150	180	8	0
Ridged BBQ Potato Chips	1 oz	150	330	10	0
Russet Valley Potato Chips	1 oz	150	180	8	0
Thin Potato Chips	1 oz	150	220	10	0
Featherweight					
Unsalted Pretzels	9 pretzels	60	15	0	0
Flavor Tree					
Fruit Nibbles Assorted	1.05 oz	120	10	2	0
Fruit Nibbles Cherry & Yogurt	1.05 oz	130	20	4	0
Fruit Nibbles Orange & Yogurt	1.05 oz	130	20	4	0
Fruit Nibbles Strawberry & Chocolate	1.05 oz	140	25	5	0
Fruit Roll Apple	1 roll	80	15	0	0
Fruit Roll Apricot	1 roll	80	15	0	0
Fruit Roll Cherry	1 roll	80	20	0	0

Brand Name	Portion	Calories	Sodium (mg)	Fat (g)	Choles. (mg)
Fruit Roll Fruit Punch	1 roll	70	10	0	0
Fruit Roll Grape	1 roll	80	15	0	0
Fruit Roll Raspberry	1 roll	80	20	0	0
Fruit Roll Strawberry	1 roll	80	10	0	0
Fritos					
BBQ Flavored Corn Chips	1 oz	150	310	9	0
King Size Dip Chips	1 oz	150	210	9	0
Fruit Corners					
Cherry Fruit Wrinkles	1 pouch	100	110	2	0
Orange Fruit Wrinkles	1 pouch	100	110	2	0
Strawberry Fruit Wrinkles	1 pouch	100	110	2	0
Watermelon Fruit Wrinkles	1 pouch	100	70	2	0
Fruit Roll-ups					
Cherry	1 roll	50	10	0	0
Fruit Punch	1 roll	50	10	0	0
Strawberry	1 roll	50	10	0	0
Watermelon	1 roll	50	10	0	0
Jolly Time					
Microwave Popcorn-Natural	3 cups	160	180	10	0
White Popcorn	4 cups	75	0	1	0
Yellow Popcorn	4 cups	88	0	1	0
Lay's					
BBQ Potato Chips	1 oz	150	340	9	0
Mr. Salty Pretzel Sticks	90 sticks	110	620	1	0
Potato Chips	1 oz	150	240	10	0
Pretzel Twists	5 twists	110	590	2	0
Unsalted Potato Chips	1 oz	150	10	10	0
Nabisco					
Veri-Thin Pretzel Sticks	45 sticks	110	770	1	0
O'Grady's					
Extra Thick Cheese Potato Chips	1 oz	150	330	8	0
Extra Thick Potato Chips	1 oz	150	210	9	0
Extra Thick Seasoned Potato Chips	1 oz	150	210	9	0
Pringle's					
Light BBQ Potato Chips	1 oz	150	125	8	0
Potato Chips, Light Style	1 oz	150	120	8	0
Regular Potato Chips	1 oz	170	170	13	0
Sour Cream & Onion Potato Chips	1 oz	170	135	12	0

Brand Name	Portion	Calories	Sodium (mg)	Fat (g)	Choles. (mg)
Snacks *cont.*					
Quaker					
Chewy Granola Bar: Nut & Raisin	1 bar	130	85	6	0
Chocolate Chip	1 bar	130	90	5	0
Granola Dips: Chewy Nut	1 bar	150	80	6	0
Peanut Butter Chocolate Chip	1 bar	130	110	6	0
Raisin/Cinnamon	1 bar	130	90	5	0
Real Fresh					
Muy Fresco Microwave Nachos	3.5 oz	140	860	9	0
Rold Gold					
Pretzel Rods	1 oz	110	520	2	0
Pretzel Sticks	1 oz	110	780	1	0
Pretzel Twists	1 oz	110	780	1	0
Tiny Tim Pretzels	1 oz	110	590	2	0
Ruffles					
Potato Chips Regular	1 oz	150	250	10	0
Potato Chips Sour Cream	1 oz	150	250	9	0
Snyder's/Hanover					
Old Fashioned Hard Pretzels	1 oz	110	650	0	0
Sunkist					
Fun Fruit Animals	0.9 oz	100	10	1	0
Fun Fruit Cherry	0.9 oz	100	10	1	0
Fun Fruit Dinosaurs	0.9 oz	100	10	1	0
Fun Fruit Grape	0.9 oz	100	10	10	0
Fun Fruit Letters	0.9 oz	100	10	1	0
Fun Fruit Numbers	0.9 oz	100	10	1	0
Fun Fruit Space Shapes	1 pouch	100	10	1	0
Fun Fruit Spooky Fruit	1 pouch	100	10	1	0
Fun Fruit Strawberry	0.9 oz	100	10	1	0
2-T-Fruit Strawberry/Cherry	1 pouch	90	25	1	0
2-T-Fruit Strawberry/Grape	1 pouch	90	25	1	0
Tostitos					
Nacho Cheese Tortilla Chips	1 oz	140	170	8	0
Traditional Flavor Tortilla Chips	1 oz	140	170	8	0
SOUPS					
Andersen's					
Cream of Potato	7.5 oz	220	790	11	0
Tomato Soup	7.5 oz	140	950	4	0
Maruchan					
Ramen Supreme Oriental Flavor	1.5 oz	200	900	8	0

Brand Name	Portion	Calories	Sodium (mg)	Fat (g)	Choles. (mg)
Nile Spice Foods					
CousCous Soup Minestrone	10.5 oz	190	625	0	0
Golden CousCous Soup Parmesan	10.5 oz	200	650	0	0
Snow's					
New England Clam Chowder	3.75 oz	70	620	2	0

SUGAR AND SUGAR SUBSTITUTES— ALL ARE CHOLESTEROL FREE

SYRUPS

Aunt Jemima					
Lite Syrup	2 tbsp	50	90	0	0
Syrup	2 tbsp	110	30	0	0
Golden Griddle					
Pancake Syrup	1 tbsp	50	15	0	0
Karo					
Dark Corn Syrup	1 tbsp	60	40	0	0
Light Corn Syrup	1 tbsp	60	30	0	0
Pancake Syrup	1 tbsp	60	35	0	0
Mrs. Butterworth					
Grandma's Molasses	1 tbsp	70	25	0	0
Grandma's Molasses—					
Green Label	1 tbsp	70	57	0	0
Lite Syrup	2 tbsp	60	65	0	0

VEGETABLES, CANNED AND FROZEN

Canned

Cara Mia					
Marinated Artichoke Crowns	1 oz	12	140	0	0
Marinated Artichoke Hearts	1 oz	27	146	2	0
Marinated Mushrooms	1 oz	13	52	1	0
Seasoned Whole Mushrooms	1 oz	7	97	0	0
Del Monte					
Asparagus Spears	½ cup	20	355	0	0
Cream-style Corn, Unsalted	½ cup	80	10	1	0
Cut Golden Wax Beans	½ cup	20	355	0	0
Cut Green Beans, No Salt Added	½ cup	20	10	0	0
French-style Green Beans, Unsalted	½ cup	20	10	0	0
French-style Green Beans	½ cup	20	355	0	0
Green Lima Beans	½ cup	70	355	0	0
Leaf Spinach, Unsalted	½ cup	25	35	0	0

Brand Name	Portion	Calories	Sodium (mg)	Fat (g)	Choles. (mg)
Del Monte cont.					
Seasoned French-style Green					
Beans	½ cup	20	355	0	0
Sliced Carrots	½ cup	30	265	0	0
Stewed Tomatoes	½ cup	35	355	0	0
Sweet Peas, No Salt Added	½ cup	60	10	0	0
Whole Green Beans	½ cup	20	355	0	0
Whole Kernel Corn, Unsalted	½ cup	80	10	1	0
Whole Peeled Tomatoes	½ cup	25	220	0	0
Zucchini in Tomato Sauce	½ cup	30	485	0	0
Dromedary					
Diced Pimientos	1 oz	10	5	0	0
Sliced Pimientos	1 oz	10	5	0	0
Dunbar's Cal-Sun					
Diced Pimientos	½ oz	4	3	0	0
Sliced Pimientos	½ oz	4	3	0	0
Green Giant					
Cream-style Corn	½ cup	100	390	1	0
Cut Asparagus	½ cup	20	420	0	0
Cut Green Beans	½ cup	20	300	0	0
Delicorn	½ cup	80	390	1	0
Diagonal-cut Green Beans	½ cup	20	280	0	0
Golden Corn	½ cup	80	310	1	0
Green Beans Almondine	½ cup	50	350	3	0
LeSueur Early Peas	½ cup	50	330	3	0
Mexicorn	½ cup	80	310	1	0
Mushroom Stems and Pieces	½ cup	25	430	0	0
Mushrooms	½ cup	25	430	0	0
Niblets Corn	½ cup	80	220	0	0
Peas & Carrots with Onions	½ cup	50	510	0	0
Sliced Mushrooms	½ cup	25	430	0	0
Sweet Peas	½ cup	50	320	0	0
White Shoepeg Corn	½ cup	90	270	0	0
3-bean Salad	½ cup	90	710	0	0
Hunt's					
Italian-style Tomato Paste	2 oz	30	—	0	0
Stewed Tomatoes, No Salt Added	4 oz	35	20	0	0
Tomato Paste	2 oz	30	—	0	0
Tomato Paste with Garlic	2 oz	30	—	0	0
Larsen's					
Veg-all Homestyle Vegetables	½ cup	35	380	0	0
Veg-all Lite Mixed Vegetables	½ cup	35	25	0	0

Brand Name	Portion	Calories	Sodium (mg)	Fat (g)	Choles. (mg)
Veg-all Mixed Vegetables	½ cup	35	320	0	0
Veg-all Peas & Carrots	½ cup	50	340	0	0
Libby's					
Bavarian-style Sauerkraut	½ cup	30	780	0	0
Cream-style Sweet Corn	½ cup	80	260	0	0
Cut Beans	½ cup	35	270	0	0
Cut Blue Lake Green Beans	½ cup	20	340	0	0
Cut Wax Beans	½ cup	20	340	0	0
Sauerkraut	½ cup	20	780	0	0
Sliced Beets	½ cup	35	270	0	0
Sliced Carrots	½ cup	20	250	0	0
Sliced Pickled Beets	½ cup	80	270	0	0
Small Whole Beets	½ cup	35	270	0	0
Sweet Peas	½ cup	60	360	0	0
Whole Green Beans	½ cup	20	340	0	0
Whole Kernel Sweet Corn	½ cup	80	360	1	0
Thank You Brand					
Cut Asparagus Spears	½ cup	20	360	0	0
Fingerling Carrots	½ cup	30	450	0	0
Whole Asparagus Spears	½ cup	25	400	0	0
Frozen					
Birds Eye					
Broccoli Cuts	⅔ cup	24	24	1	0
Classic Corn in Butter	½ cup	62	43	1	0
Corn on the Cob	1 ear	156	4	1	0
Corn, Whole Kernel Cut	½ cup	82	3	1	0
Cut Green Beans	½ cup	24	3	1	0
Deluxe Tiny Tender Peas	½ cup	62	118	1	0
Farm Fresh Broccoli/Cauliflower/ Carrots	⅔ cup	26	26	1	0
Farm Fresh Broccoli/Red Peppers/ Bamboo Shoots	⅔ cup	23	16	1	0
Farm Fresh Brussels Sprouts/ Cauliflower/Carrots	⅔ cup	31	20	1	0
Farm Fresh Cauliflower/Carrots/ Snow Peas	⅔ cup	30	26	1	0
Fresh Green Beans with Almonds	½ cup	51	335	2	0
Green Peas	½ cup	76	132	1	0
Mixed Vegetables	½ cup	62	43	1	0
Peas & Pearl Onions	½ cup	139	482	7	0
Rice & Peas with Mushrooms	⅔ cup	108	322	1	0

Brand Name	Portion	Calories	Sodium (mg)	Fat (g)	Choles. (mg)
Birds Eye cont.					
Small Whole Onions	½ cup	40	10	0	0
C & W					
Chinese Pea Pods	3½ oz	43	5	0	0
Chinese Pea Pods with Water					
Chestnuts	3½ oz	59	5	0	0
Parisienne Carrots	3½ oz	37	42	0	0
Petite Green Peas	3½ oz	74	150	0	0
Petite Sweet Corn	3½ oz	79	1	1	0
Ore-Ida					
Cob Corn	1 ear	180	40	2	0
Golden Crinkles	3 oz	120	35	4	0
Golden Fries	3 oz	120	35	4	0
Home Style Potato Wedges	3 oz	100	45	3	0
Microwave Hash Browns	2 oz	130	170	8	0
Microwave Tater Tots	4 oz	200	670	9	0
Potatoes O'Brien	3 oz	60	25	0	0
Shredded Hash Browns	3 oz	70	40	0	0
Southern Style Hash Browns	3 oz	70	35	0	0
Pictsweet					
Broccoli Cuts	3.2 oz	25	25	0	0
California Blend	3.2 oz	25	20	0	0
Cut Corn	3.2 oz	101	0	1	0
Green Peas	3.2 oz	80	110	1	0
Mixed Vegetables	3.2 oz	60	60	0	0
Vegetables Del Sol	3.2 oz	30	35	0	0
Vegetables Grande	3.2 oz	45	15	0	0
Vegetables Japanese	3.2 oz	25	10	0	0
Vegetables Milano	3.2 oz	40	40	0	0
Stokely					
Singles Broccoli/Carrots					
Water Chestnuts	3 oz	30	22	1	0
Singles Broccoli/Cauliflower	3 oz	20	15	1	0
Singles Broccoli/Cauliflower/					
Carrots	3 oz	25	25	1	0
Singles Cut Corn	3 oz	75	5	1	0

BIBLIOGRAPHIC
NOTES

T hese notes contain references to the studies mentioned in the text as well as to the large body of medical literature that forms the groundwork on which this book stands.

For purposes of brevity, associate authors are not listed.

CHAPTER 1: HEART DISEASE CAN BE REVERSED

"Dietary fat and its relation to heart attacks and strokes," J Amer Med Assn, Special Communications, Feb. 4, 1961.

L. Aschoff, "Atherosclerosis." In Lectures in Pathology. New York: Hoeber, 1924.

W. Raab, "Dietary factors in the origin of arteriosclerosis and hypertension." In Prevention of Ischemic Heart Disease. Springfield, IL: Charles C. Thomas.

A Farewell to Heart Disease

H. E. Schornagel, "The connection between nutrition and mortality from coronary sclerosis during and after World War II," Documenta Medicina Geographica Trophica, 5, 1953.

A. Strom, "Mortality from circulatory disease in Norway 1940–45," Lancet, Jan. 20, 1951.

I. Vartianen, "Report on Finland," Ann Med Int Fenniae, 36, 1957.

G. Schettler, Report at Symposium on Coronary Artery Disease, New York Academy of Sciences, Oct. 1961.

G. Schettler, "Cardiovascular disease during and after World War II: A comparison of the Federal Republic of Germany with other European countries," Preventive Med, 8, 1979.

F. A. Pezold, Arteriosclerosis and Nutrition, Steinkopf, Germany, 1959.

How Atherosclerosis Builds

C. M. W. Adams, "A hypothesis to explain the accumulation of cholesterol in atherosclerosis," Lancet, April 28, 1962.

W. F. Enos, "Coronary disease among United States soldiers killed in action in Korea," J Amer Med Assn, July 18, 1953.

T. R. Dawber, "The epidemiology of coronary heart disease: The Framingham Enquiry," Proc R Soc Med, 55, 1962.

J. Stamler, "Atherosclerotic coronary heart disease—etiology and pathogenesis: The epidemiologic findings." In Lectures on Preventive Cardiology. New York: Grune & Stratton, 1967.

D. H. Blankenhorn, "The prevention, declaration, and possible regression of coronary atherosclerosis. In Update III: The Heart. New York: McGraw Hill, 1980.

R. H. Heptinstall, "Relative roles of blood cholesterol level and blood pressure level in the production of experimental aortic atheroma in rabbits," Angiology, 9, 1958.

K. W. Walton, "The evolution of human atherosclerotic lesions." In Regression of Atherosclerotic Lesions: Experimental Studies and Observations in Humans, (ed) M. René Malinow. New York: Plenum Press, 1984.

Berenson and Lauer information from Cardiovascular Research Reports, Number 31, Summer 1989. "Evidence from Bogalusa: Heart disease starts in childhood," page 8.

"Seeing" Reversal

D. Rutstein, "Effects of linolenic and stearic acids on cholesterol-induced lipoid deposition in human aortic cells in tissue culture," Lancet, March 15, 1958.

S. L. Wilens, "Resorption of arterial atheromatous deposits in wasting disease," Amer J Pathol, 23, 1947.

M. R. Malinow, "Arterial pathology in cancer patients suggests atherosclerosis regression," Med Hypotheses, 11, 1983.

M. R. Malinow, "Atherosclerosis: Progression, regression and resolution," Amer Heart J, 108, 1984.

Direct Observation on Animals

I. Anitschkow, "A history of experimentation on arterial atherosclerosis in animals." In Arteriosclerosis: A Survey of the Problem. New York: Macmillan, 1933.

K. E. Fritz, "Regression of advanced atherosclerosis in swine," Arch Pathol Lab Med, 100, 1967.

R. W. Wissler, "Interaction of therapeutic diets and cholesterol-lowering drugs in regression studies in animals." In Regression of Atherosclerotic Lesions: Experimental Studies and Observations in Humans, NATO Series. New York: Plenum Press, 1984.

G. DePalma, "Approaches to evaluating regression of experimental atherosclerosis," Adv Exp Med Biol, 1977.

M. R. Malinow, "Plant Glycosides: Effects on atherosclerosis regression in macaca fascicularis." In Regression of Atherosclerotic Lesions: Experimental Studies and Observations in Humans, NATO Series. New York: Plenum Press, 1984.

M. R. Malinow, "Effect of alfalfa meal on shrinkage (regression) of atherosclerotic plaque during cholesterol feeding in monkeys," Atherosclerosis, 30, 1978.

M. R. Malinow, "Regression of atherosclerosis in humans: Fact or myth?," Circulation, 64, 1981.

M. R. Malinow, "Regression in nonhuman primates," Circulation Res, 46, 1980.

D. H. Blankenhorn, "Angiography for study of lipid-lowering therapy," Circulation, 59, 1979.

M. Miller, "Lipid abnormalities in coronary disease patients with 'desirable' cholesterol levels: Should we screen all CAD patients for low HDL levels?" Abstract 1525. 61st Scientific Sessions of the American Heart Association.

D. H. Blankenhorn, "Lipoproteins and the progression and regression of atherosclerosis," Cardiovascular Reviews and Reports, 3, 1982.

D. Roth, "Non-invasive and invasive demonstration of spontaneous regression of coronary artery disease," Circulation, 62, 1980.

H. Buckwald, "Surgical treatment of hyperlipidemia," Circulation, 49, 1974.

L. Knight, "Radiographic appraisal of the Minnesota partial ileal bypass," Surg Form, 23, 1972.

R. I. Levy, "The influence of changes in lipid values induced by cholestyramine and diet on progression of coronary artery disease," Circulation, 69, 1984.

D. M. Ornish, "Can lifestyle changes reverse atherosclerosis?," Circulation, 78, 1988.

R. Barndt, Jr., "Regression and progression of early femoral atherosclerosis in treated hyperlipoproteinemic patients," Ann Intern Med, 86, 1977.

W. Rafflenbeul, "Quantitative coronary arteriography: Coronary anatomy of patients with unstable angina pectoris re-examined 1 year after optimal medical therapy," Amer J Cardiology, 43, 1979.

M. R. Malinow, "Regression of atherosclerosis in humans: Anatomical evidence from postmortem studies." In Regression of Atherosclerotic Lesions: Experimental Studies and Observations in Humans, (ed) M. René Malinow. New York: Plenum Press, 1984.

W. Wartman, "The incidence of heart disease in 2,000 consecutive autopsies," Ann Intern Med, 28, 1948.

K. Horlick, "Retrogression of atherosclerotic lesions on cessation of cholesterol feeding in the chick," J Lab Clin Med, 34, 1949.

M. J. Jesse, "Task force 1: The physician and children (pediatric and adolescent practice and the school)." The Bethesda Conference: Prevention of Coronary Heart Disease, Amer J Cardiology, 47, 1981.

A joint statement for physicians . . . "Diagnosis and treatment of primary hyperlipidemia in childhood," American Heart Association, 1986.

CHAPTER 2: THE REVERSAL DIET PROGRAM

W. B. Kannel, "Epidemiology of heart disease: Epidemiological insights into atherosclerotic cardiovascular disease." In Heart Disease and Rehabilitation, (ed) Pollack & Schmidt. Boston: Houghton Mifflin Professional Publishers, 1979.

When Will Reversal Take Place?

H. C. Stary, "Progression and regression of experimental atherosclerosis in rhesus monkeys." In Medical Primatology. Basel: S. Karger, 1972.

M. L. Armstrong, "Regression of coronary atheromatosis in rhesus monkeys," Circ. Res., 38, 1976.

D. M. Kramsch, "Reduction of coronary atherosclerosis by moderate conditioning exercise in monkeys on an atherogenic diet," New Eng J Med, 305, 1981.

A. G. Olsson, "Regression of computer estimated femoral atherosclerosis after pronounced serum lipid lowering in patients with asymptomatic hyperlipidemia," Lancet, 1, 1982.

D. W. Crawford, "Computer densitometry for angiographic assessment of arterial cholesterol content and gross pathology in human atherosclerosis," J Lab Clin Med, 89, 1977.

R. G. M. Duffield, "Treatment of hyperlipidemia retards progression of symptomatic femoral atherosclerosis: A random controlled trial," Lancet, 1, 1983.

K. Cohn, "Effect of clofibrate on progression of coronary disease: A prospective angiographic study in man," Amer Heart J, 89, 1975.

J. F. Brensike, "Effects of therapy with cholestyramine on progression of coronary arteriosclerosis: Results of the NHLBI Type II Coronary Intervention Study," Circulation, 69, 1984.

K. M. Detre, "Secondary prevention and lipid lowering: Results and implications," Amer Heart J, 110, 1985.

A. C. Arntzenius, "Diet, lipoproteins, and the progression of coronary atherosclerosis: The Leiden Intervention Trial," New Eng J Med, 312, 1985.

D. Roth, "Noninvasive and invasive demonstration of spontaneous regression of coronary artery disease," Circulation, 62, 1980.

R. G. DePalma, "Progression and regression of experimental atherosclerosis," Surg Gynecol Obstet, 131, 1970.

D. H. Blankenhorn, "Blood cholesterol levels and atherosclerosis regression," Cardiology Board Review, 6 (suppl.), 1989.

Goal 1: To Reduce Cholesterol

K. Anderson, "Cholesterol and mortality: 30 years of follow-up from the Framingham Study," J Amer Med Assn, 257, no. 16, 1987.
G. Assmann, "High-density lipoproteins and their role in preventing or retarding atherosclerosis." In Regression of Atherosclerotic Lesions: Experimental Studies and Observations in Humans, (ed) M. René Malinow. New York: Plenum Press, 1984.

The dietary goals of the Reversal Diet Program are based largely upon the Step 1 guidelines established by the National Cholesterol Education Program (NCEP) which are based upon the following studies:

United States Department of Agriculture. Human Nutrition Information Service. "Dietary guidelines for Americans," DHHS, Home and Garden Bulletin, 232, 1986.
S. M. Grundy, "Rationale of the diet-heart statement of the American Heart Association." Report of the Nutrition Committee, Circulation, 65, 1982.
J. Stamler, "Population studies." In Nutrition, Lipids, and Coronary Disease: A Global View. New York: Raven, 1979.
I. Hjermann, "Effect of diet and smoking intervention on the incidence of coronary heart disease," Lancet, 2, 1981.
A. M. Gotto, "Recommendations for treatment of hyperlipidemia in adults." A joint statement of the Nutrition Committee and the Council on Arteriosclerosis. Circulation, 69, 1984.
A. Keys, "Serum cholesterol response to changes in the diet," Metabolism, 14, 1965.
D. M. Hegsted, "Quantitative effects of dietary fat on serum cholesterol in man," Amer J Clin Nutr, 27, 1974.
A. Keys, "Bias and misrepresentation revisited: Perspective on saturated fat," Amer J Clin Nutr, 27, 1974.
A. Keys, "Coronary heart disease in seven countries," Circulation, 41 (suppl. I), 1970.
P. M. Herold, "Fish oil consumption and decreased risk of cardiovascular disease: A comparison of findings from animal and human feeding trials," Amer J Clin Nutr, 43, 1986.
F. H. Mattson, "Effects of dietary cholesterol on serum cholesterol in man," Amer J Clin Nutr, 25, 1972.
H. Ginsberg, "Lipoprotein metabolism in nonresponders to increased dietary cholesterol," Arteriosclerosis, 1, 1981.
A. Keys, "Serum cholesterol response to dietary cholesterol," Amer J Clin Nutr, 40, 1984.
G. Schonfeld, "Effects of dietary cholesterol and fatty acids on plasma lipoproteins," Amer J Clin Invest, 69, 1982.

L. W. Anderson, "Hypocholesterolemic effects of oat-bran or bean intake for hypercholesterolemic men," Amer J Clin Nutr, 40, 1984.

W. R. Harlan, "Blood pressure and nutrition in adults: The National Health and Nutrition Examination Survey," Amer J Epidemiol, 40, 1984.

C. H. Hennekens, "Alcohol." In Prevention of Coronary Heart Disease, (ed) N. M. Kaplan & J. Stamler. Philadelphia: W. B. Saunders, 1983.

H. B. Hubert, "Obesity as an independent risk factor for cardiovascular disease: A 26-year follow-up of participants in the Framingham Heart Study," Circulation, 67, 1983.

R. B. Shekelle, "Diet, serum cholesterol, and death from coronary heart disease—The Western Electric Study," New Eng J Med, 304, 1981.

D. Kromhout, "The inverse reaction between fish consumption and 20-year mortality from coronary heart disease," New Eng J Med, 312, 1985.

American Heart Association. "Dietary guidelines for healthy American adults: A statement for physicians and health professionals by the Nutrition Committee, American Heart Association," Circulation, 74, 1986.

C. Raab, Heart to Heart: A Manual on Nutrition Counseling for the Reduction of Cardiovascular Disease Risk Factors," NIH, PHS, DHHS, NIH Pub. No. 83-1528.

United States Department of Agriculture. Human Nutrition Information Service. "Nutritive Value of Foods," Home & Garden Bulletin, no. 72, 1986.

Goal 2: Achieve a Normal Blood Pressure

The blood-pressure guidelines of the Reversal Diet Program are based on the dietary studies mentioned in this section, my own research—some of which is included in the papers cited below—and the work of others which are listed in the entries that follow.

T. A. Miettinen, "Multifactorial primary prevention of cardiovascular disease in middle-aged men," J Amer Med Assn, 254, 1985.

J. E. Manson, "Body weight and longevity: A reassessment," J Amer Med Assn, 257, 1987.

1988 Joint National Committee, "The 1988 report of the Joint National Committee on detection, evaluation, and treatment of high blood pressure," Arch Intern Med, 148, 1988.

Panel discussion, "Risk factors in heart disease," Med World News, 18, 1977.

Consensus conference, "Lowering blood cholesterol to prevent heart disease," J Amer Med Assn, 254, 1985.

J. Stamler, "Primary prevention of coronary heart disease: The last 20 years." The Bethesda Conference: Prevention of Coronary Heart Disease. Amer J Cardiology, 47, 1981.

Goal 3: Burn at Least 150 to 300 Calories a Day

The exercise guidelines are based on my own research as well as on the following studies and sources.

American College of Sports Medicine, "Position statement on the recommended quantity and quality of exercise for developing and maintaining fitness in healthy adults," Med & Sci in Sports, 10, 1978.

P. O. Astrand, Textbook of Work Physiology. New York: McGraw-Hill, 1977.

N. B. Oldridge, "Compliance and drop-out in cardiac exercise rehabilitation," J Cardiac Rehab, 4, 1984.

M. L. Pollock, Exercise Prescription for Rehabilitation of the Cardiac Patient, (ed) M. L. Pollock & D. H. Schmidt. New York: John Wiley.

Department of Health and Human Services, "Promoting health/preventing disease: Objective for the nation," Washington, DC: US Government Printing Office, 1988.

W. B. Kannel, "Some health benefits of physical activity: The Framingham Study," Arch Intern Med, 139, 1979.

W. P. Morgan, "Psychological effects of exercise," Behav Med Update, 4, 1982.

J. N. Morris, "Vigorous exercise in leisure-time: Protection against coronary heart disease," Lancet, 8206, 1980.

R. Sylvester, "Effects of exercise training on progression of documented coronary arteriosclerosis." In the Marathon: physiological, medical, epidemiological and psychological studies. (Ed) Milvy, P. Ann NY, 301, Acad Sci, 1977.

National Center for Health Statistics, "Exercise and participation in sports among persons 20 years of age or over, United States," 1975, Washington, DC: US Government Printing Office.

N. Sarkas, "Reduced fibrinolytic activity of atherosclerotic sera caused by an increase in low-density lipoproteins in blood," Nature, March 18, 1961.

R. S. Paffenbarger, "Work activity and coronary heart mortality," New Eng J Med, 292, 1975.

R. S. Paffenbarger, "Exercise in the prevention of coronary heart disease," Preventive Med, 13, 1984.

R. S. Paffenbarger, "Physical activity as an index of heart attack risk in college alumni," Amer J Epidemiol, 108, 1978.

R. Paffenbarger, "Physical activity, all-cause mortality, and longevity of college alumni," New Eng J Med, 314, 1986.

H. Blackburn, "Physical activity and the risk of coronary heart disease," New Eng J Med, 319, 1988.

L. G. Ekelund, "Physical fitness as a predictor of cardiovascular mortality in asymptomatic North American men," New Eng J Med, 319, 1988.

L. Goldberg, "Changes in lipid and lipoprotein levels after weight training," J Amer Med Assn, 252, 1984.

B. F. Hurley, "High-density-lipoprotein cholesterol in bodybuilders vs powerlifters," J Amer Med Assn, 252, 1984.

J. H. Billings, "How to help cardiac patients reduce risk factors," Physician & Sportsmedicine, 17, Sept. 1989.

R. S. Paffenbarger, Jr., "Comments on nutrition, fitness and health," A talk given at the Center for Health Communications at the Harvard School of Public Health, Jan. 16, 1987.

"Conference on exercise in the elderly: Its role in prevention of physical decline and in rehabilitation," NIH, Oct. 27–28, 1977.

S. P. Sady, "Prolonged exercise augments plasma triglyceride clearance," J Amer Med Assn, 256, 1986.

W. Raab (ed), Prevention of Ischemic Heart Disease." Springfield, IL: Charles C. Thomas.

A. S. Leon, "Leisure-time physical activity levels and risk of coronary heart disease and death: The multiple risk factor intervention trial," J Amer Med Assn, 258, 1987.

R. K. Dishman, "Mental health." In Physical Activity & Well-being, (ed) Vern Seefeldt. National Association for Sports and Physical Education, 1986.

W. Raab, "Loafer's heart," Arch Intern Med, Feb. 1958.

Goal 4: Maintain a Normal Body Weight

The body-weight guidelines are based on my own studies, the work cited in the text, and the following papers:

L. E. Manson, "Body weight and longevity: A reassesment," J Amer Med Assn, 257, 1987.

T. B. Van Itallie, "Obesity: Adverse effects on health and longevity," Am J Clin Nutr, 32, 1979.

A. Keys, "Overweight, obesity, coronary heart disease and mortality," Nutr Rev, 38, 1980.

A. Keys, "Is overweight a risk factor for coronary heart disease?," Cardiovascular Med, 1979.

T. A. Miettinen, "Multifactorial primary prevention of cardiovascular disease in middle-aged men," J Amer Med Assn, 254, 1985.

Goal 5: De-Stress Your Life

Stress guidelines were formulated from my own research, work cited in the text, and the studies mentioned below.

M. Friedman, Type A Behavior and Your Heart. New York: Alfred A. Knopf, 1974.

R. S. Eliot, "Task force 3: The physician in the work setting (Industrial/occupational medicine)," The Bethesda Conference: Prevention of Coronary Heart Disease, Amer J Cardiology, 47, 1981.

C. C. Tennant, "Anger and other psychological factors in coronary atherosclerosis," Psycholog Med, 17, 1987.

A. H. Mann, "Psychiatric morbidity and hostility in hypertension," Psycholog Med, 7, 1977.

R. B. Shekelle, "Hostility, risk of coronary heart disease and mortality," Psychosom Med, 45, 1983.

C. C. Tennant, "Psychological correlates of coronary heart disease," Psycholog Med, 15, 1985.

S. J. Zyzanski, "Psychological correlates of coronary angiographic findings," Arch Intern Med, 136, 1976.

H. K. Hellerstein, "Occupational stress, law school hierarchy, and coronary artery disease in Cleveland attorneys," Circulation (suppl. II), 31, 1966.

H. K. Hellerstein, "Behavior patterns and serum cholesterol in patent attorneys," Circulation (suppl. II), 31, 1966.

E. H. Friedman, "Coronary risk factors and the socioeconomic hierarchy in a group of middle-aged businessmen," Circulation (suppl. III), 33, 1966.

H. K. Hellerstein, "Stress and heart disease." Heart and Industry Symposium. Sheraton Boston Hotel, Nov. 9, 1967.

E. H. Friedman, "Coronary risk factors, the socioeconomic hierarchy and the control of aggression in a group of middle-aged business men," Circulation (suppl. II), 36, 1966.

E. H. Friedman, "Occupational stress, law school hierarchy and coronary artery disease in Cleveland attorneys," Psychosom Med, 30, 1968.

E. H. Friedman, "Behavior patterns and serum cholesterol in two groups of normal males," Amer J Med Sci, 255, 1968.

Goal 6: Use No Tobacco

The smoking guidelines came from my own work, the studies mentioned in the text, and the papers cited below.

1988 Joint National Committee, "The 1988 report of the Joint National Committee on detection, evaluation, and treatment of high blood pressure," Arch Intern Med, 148, 1988.

B. Schucker, "Changes in physician perspective on cholesterol and heart disease: Results from two national surveys," J Amer Med Assn, 258, 1987.

T. Miettinen, "Multifactorial primary prevention of cardiovascular diseases in middle-aged men: Risk factor changes, incidence and mortality," J Amer Med Assn, 254, 1985.

I. Hjermann, "Effects of diet and smoking intervention on the incidence of coronary heart disease: Report from the Oslo study group of a randomized trial in healthy men," Lancet, 2, 1981.

Multiple Risk Factor Intervention Trial Research Group, "Multiple risk factor intervention trial: Risk factor changes and mortality results," J Amer Med Assn, 248, 1982.

K. A. Perkins, "The effect of nicotine on energy expenditure during light physical activity," New Eng J Med, 320, 1989.

J. Barry, "Effect of smoking on the activity of ischemic heart disease," J Amer Med Assn, 261, 1989.

Health consequences of smoking: Cardiovascular Disease. A Report from the Surgeon General. US Dept of Health and Human Services, 1983.

J. D. Folts, "The effects of cigarette smoke and nicotine on platelet thrombus formation in stenosed dog coronary arteries," Circulation, 65, 1982.

H. Schievelbein, "Cardiovascular action of nicotine and smoking," JNCI, 48, 1974.

R. J. Garrison, "Cigarette smoking and HDL cholesterol: The Framingham offspring study," Atherosclerosis, 30, 1978.

J. L. Martin, "Acute coronary vasoconstriction effects of cigarette smoking in coronary heart disease," Am J Cardiology, 54, 1984.

N. A. Rigotti, "Cigarette smoking and body weight," New Eng J Med, 320, 1989.

J. F. Doyle, "Cigarette smoking and coronary disease," New Eng J Med, April 19, 1962.

Goal 7: Maintain Normal Blood-Sugar Levels

Blood-sugar guidelines came from work cited in the text, my own research, and the studies that are listed below.

"Report of the national Cholesterol Education Program Expert Panel on Detection, Evaluation, and Treatment of High Blood Cholesterol in Adults," Arch Intern Med, 148, 1988.

Working group on hypertension in diabetes, "Statement on hypertension in diabetes mellitus: final report," Arch Intern Med, 147, 1987.

H. C. Simpson, "A high carbohydrate leguminous fiber diet improves all aspects of diabetic control," Lancet, 1, 1981.

I. M. Liebow, "Cardiac complications of diabetes mellitus," Amer J Med, 7, 1949.

I. M. Liebow, "Arteriosclerotic heart disease in diabetes mellitus," Circulation, 4, 1951.

I. M. Liebow, "Arteriosclerotic heart disease in diabetes mellitus." A clinical study. Proc. 27th Sc. Sess., American Heart Association, 50, 1954.

I. M. Liebow, "Arteriosclerotic heart disease in diabetes mellitus. A clinical study of 383 patients," Amer J Med, 18, 1955.

1988 Joint National Committee, "The 1988 report of the Joint National Committee on detection, evaluation, and treatment of high blood pressure," Arch Intern Med, 148, May 1988.

G. Reaven, "Glucose tolerance in patients with myocardial infarction," American Heart Association, Oct. 1962.

"Coronary risk factor statement for the American public," American Heart Association, Pamphlet, 1987.

"Killing two risks with one diet." Article on Jeremiah Stamler study of eating habits of 519 men with two or more risk factors for heart disease, Med World News, 18, 1977.

T. Leary. Arch Pathol, April 1936.

CHAPTER 3: YOUR REVERSAL PROFILE

The seven-day diary used in this chapter is a variation of diaries that I have used in studies and with individual patients. Other portions of the text in this chapter came from my own experiences and the facts imparted by the following studies:

"Report of the national Cholesterol Education Program Expert Panel on Detection, Evaluation, and Treatment of High Blood Cholesterol in Adults," Arch Intern Med, 148, 1988.

"Current status of blood cholesterol measurement in clinical laboratories in the United States: A report from the Laboratory Standardization Panel of the National Cholesterol Education Program," Clin Chem, 34, 1988.

H. K. Naito, "Reliability of lipid and lipoprotein testing," Amer J Cardiology, 56, 1985.

H. K. Naito, "The ABC's of cholesterol standardization," College of American Pathologists, 1988.

R. Stamler, "Primary prevention of hypertension by nutritional-hygenic means," J Amer Med Assn, 262, Oct. 6, 1989.

R. Stamler, "Nutritional therapy for high blood pressure: Final report of a four-year randomized controlled trial—The Hypertension Control Program," J Amer Med Assn, 257, 1987.

J. Stamler, "Lifestyles, major risk factors, proof and public policy," Circulation, 58, 1978.

S. M. Grundy, "Rationale of the diet-heart statement of the American Heart Association: Report of the Nutrition Committee," Circulation, 65, 1982.

S. M. Grundy, "Coronary disease: The lipoprotein connection," Cardiology, Jan. 1984.

CHAPTER 4: GETTING THE LEAD OUT

Most of the advice in this chapter comes from years of helping patients make meaningful life-style changes. It is commonly accepted advice in the world of preventive cardiology. Other information that draws on the research of others is duly cited in the text.

CHAPTER 5: DEFENSIVE EATING

In addition to studies cited in the text, here are some of the studies that formed the groundwork for this chapter:

A. Keys, Seven Countries: A Multivariate Analysis of Death and Coronary Heart Disease. Cambridge, MA: Harvard University Press, 1980.

D. P. Burkitt, "Dietary fiber and disease," J Amer Med Assn, 229, 1974.

D. P. Burkitt, "Etiology and prevention of colorectal cancer," Hospital Practice, February 1984.

G. Goldsmith. Arch Intern Med, April 1960.

C. J. Glueck, "Appraisal of dietary fat as a causative factor in atherogenesis," Amer J Clin Nutr, 32, 1979.

C. J. Glueck, "Dietary fat and atherosclerosis," Amer J Clin Nutr, 32, 1979.

M. R. Malinow, "Plant glycosides: Effects on atherosclerosis regression in macaca fascicularis." In Regression of Atherosclerotic Lesions: Experimental Studies and Observations in Humans," (ed) M. R. Malinow and V. H. Blaton. New York: Plenum Press, 1984.

J. Swain, "Comparison of the effects of oat bran and low-fiber wheat on serum lipoprotein levels and blood pressure," New Eng J Med, 332, Jan. 18, 1990.

W. E. Connors, "Dietary fiber—nostrom or critical nutrient?," New Eng J Med, 332, Jan. 18, 1990.

Proving Fiber

D. H. Blankenhorn, "The cholesterol lowering atherosclerosis study," J Amer Med Assn, June 19, 1987.

M. Burros, "Oat bran: The muffin and the mania." New York Times, Oct. 26, 1988, Section C-1.

E. G. Knox, "Food and disease," Brit J Prev Soc Med, 31, 1977.

A. Keys, "Serum cholesterol response to changes in diet." Parts 1–5, Metabolism, 14, 1965.

J. C. Witteman, "Dietary calcium and magnesium and hypertension: a prospective study." Circulation, 1987, 76.

D. A. McCarron, "Blood pressure and nutrient intake in the United States," Science, 1984, 224.

D. M. Hegsted, "Quantitative effect of dietary factors on serum cholesterol in man," Amer J Clin Nutr, 17, 1965.

M. Stasse-Wolthuis, "The effect of a natural high-fiber on serum lipids, fecal lipids and colonic function," Amer J Clin Nutr, 32, 1979.

P. D. White, "Survey of cardiovascular disease among Africans in the vicinity of the Albert Schweitzer Hospital in 1960," Amer J Cardiology, Sept. 1962.

K. L. Chi, "Cardiovascular diseases in China," Amer J Cardiology, Sept. 1962.

P. E. Steiner, Arch Path, October 1946.

H. C. Trowell, "A case of coronary heart disease in an African," East African Med J, October 1956.

L. Kiang, "Dietary lipids, sugar, fiber, and mortality from coronary heart disease: Bivariate analysis of international data," Arteriosclerosis, 2, 1982.

J. Groen, "The influence of nutrition, individuality and some other factors, including various forms of stress, on the serum cholesterol," Voeding, Nov. 1952.

D. P. Burkitt, "Etiology and prevention of colorectal cancer," Hospital Practice, February 1984.

J. W. Anderson, "Hypocholesterolemic effects of oat bran for hypercholesterolemic men," Am J Clin Nutr, 1981, 34.

J. W. Anderson, "Hypocholesterolemic effects of high fibre diets rich in water-soluble plant fibres," J Can Diet Assoc, 1984, 45.

The Friendly Fin

D. Kromhout, "The inverse relation between fish consumption and 20-year mortality from coronary heart disease," New Eng J Med, 19, 1985.

B. E. Phillipson, "Reduction of plasma lipids, lipoproteins, and apoproteins by dietary fish oils in patients with hypertriglyceridemia," N Eng J Med, 312, 1985.

W. P. Singer, "Clinical studies on lipid and blood pressure lowering effect of eicosapentaenoic acid-rich diet," Biomed Bimchim Acta, 43, 1984.

P. G. Noms, "Effect of dietary supplementation with fish oil on systolic blood pressure in mild essential hypertension," Brit Med J, 293, 1986.

M. Milner, "High dose Omega-3 fatty acid supplementation reduces clinical restenosis after coronary angioplasty," 61st Scientific Session of the American Heart Association, Abstract 2527.

T. H. Lee, "Effect of dietary enrichment with eicosapentaenoic and docosahexaenoic acids on in vitro neutrophil and monocyte leukotriene generation and neutrophil function," New Eng J Med, 19, 1985.

J. A. Glomset, "Fish, fatty acids, and human health," New Eng J Med, 19, 1985.

J. Dyerberg, "Plasma lipid and lipoprotein pattern in Greenlandic west-coast Eskimos," Lancet, 1, 1971.

T. O. Lossonczy, "The effect of a fish diet on serum lipids in healthy human subjects," Amer J Clin Nutr, 31, 1978.

W. S. Harris, "The comparative reductions of the plasma lipids and lipoproteins by dietary polyunsaturated fats: Salmon oil vs vegetable oils," Metabolism, 32, 1983.

A. M. Fehily, "The effect of fatty fish on plasma lipid and lipoprotein concentrations," Amer J Clin Nutr, 38, 1983.

S. H. Goodnight, "Polyunsaturated fatty acids, hyperlipidemia, and thrombosis," Arteriosclerosis, 2, 1982.

J. Exler, "Finfish: Comprehensive evaluation of fatty acids in foods," J Amer Diet Assn, 69, 1976.

W. S. Harris, "The effects of salmon oil upon plasma lipids, lipoproteins and triglycerides clearance," Trans Assn Amer Physicians, 43, 1980.

J. H. Rapp, "Lipids of human atherosclerotic plaques and xanthomas: Clues to the mechanism of plaque regression," J Lipid Res, 24, 1983.

P. J. Nestel, "Suppression by diets rich in fish oil of very low density lipoprotein production in man," J Clin Invest, 74, 1984.

D. R. Illingworth, "Inhibition of low density lipoprotein to low density lipoprotein synthesis by dietary Omega-3 fatty acids in humans," Arteriosclerosis, 4, 1984.

F. P. Zeller, "Fish oil: Effectiveness as a dietary supplement in the prevention of heart disease," Drug Intelligence & Clin Phar, 21, July/Aug 1987.

. . . And More Defensive Foods

W. Castelli, "Alcohol and blood lipids," Lancet, 2, 1977.

N. Ernst, "The association of plasma HDL cholesterol with dietary intake and alcohol consumption," Circulation, 62 (suppl.), 1980.

J. Thornton, "Moderate alcohol intake reduces bile cholesterol saturation and raises HDL cholesterol," Lancet, 2, 1983.

T. Turner, "The beneficial side of moderate alcohol use," Johns Hopkins Med J, 148, 1981.

A. Bordia, "Effects of garlic feeding on regression of experimental atherosclerosis in rabbits," Artery, 7, 1980.

T. Ariga, "Platelet aggregation inhibitor in garlic," Lancet, 1, 1981.

R. Arora, "Comparative effect of clofibrate, garlic and onion on alimentary hyperlipidemia," Atherosclerosis, 39, 1981.

D. Boullin, "Garlic as a platelet inhibitor," Lancet, 1, 1981.

CHAPTER 6: ON THE ROAD

Most of the advice in this chapter comes from years of helping patients make meaningful life-style changes. Much of it is commonly accepted advice in the world of preventive cardiology, while other portions of it come from my attempts and those of my co-author to live on the road in a sometimes heart-hostile world. Information that draws on the research of others is duly cited in the text. Here is some of the research that helped form the groundwork for this chapter.

"Modify your behavior to keeps pounds off!," Choices in Cardiol, 3, 1989.

C. Roberts, "Sounding board: Fast food fare," New Eng J Med, 321, 1989.

M. Sheridan, Fast Food and the American Diet. New York: American Council on Science and Health, 1983.

Department of Health and Human Services, The Surgeon General's Report on Nutrition and Health: Summary and Recommendations 1988. Washington, DC: US Government Printing Office, 1988.

S. M. Grundy, "Rationale of the diet-heart statement of the American Heart Association: Report of Nutritional Committee," Circulation, 65, 1982.

D. J. A. Jenkins, "Nibbling versus gorging: Metabolic advantages of increased meal frequency," New Eng J Med, 321, 1989.

C. Cohn, "Feeding frequency and protein metabolism," Amer J Physiol, 205, 1963.

CHAPTER 7: EXERCISE

This chapter combines personal experience, studies cited in Chapter 2 in "Goal 3," and my own studies on exercise which are cited below:

H. K. Hellerstein, "Returning sick hearts to work," Proc. Heart in Industry Conf., Chicago Heart Assn, 17, 1952.

H. K. Hellerstein, "Electrocardiographic exercise to tolerance tests in old myocardial infarction," J Lab & Clin Med, 40, 1952.

E. M. Kline, "Heart disease and industrial medicine: The placement, protection and rehabilitation of persons suffering from heart disease," Indust Med, 22, 1953.

H. K. Hellerstein, "Work classification clinic of the heart society," Bulletin Acad Med, Cleveland, 12, 1953.

H. K. Hellerstein, "Rehabilitation of patients with heart disease," Postgrad Med 15, 1954.

H. K. Hellerstein, "Outlook for cardiacs: Experience of the Cleveland Work Classification Clinic Program Part II," Second World Congress of Cardiology, Washington, DC, Sept. 12, 1954.

T. W. Moir, "Team approach in rehabilitating the cardiac patient. Experience of the Cleveland Work Classification Clinic," Ohio's Health, 8, 1958.

L. N. Katz, "Rehabilitation of the cardiac patient (panel discussion)," Circulation, 17, 1958.

A. B. Ford, "Work and heart disease: A physiologic study in the factory," Circulation, 18, 1958.

D. J. Turrell, "Six year average follow-up of 460 consecutive cardiac patients," Circulation, 18, 1958.

H. K. Hellerstein, "Work load and cardiac function," Conf. Heart Ind. NY Heart Assn, 25, 1959.

H. K. Hellerstein, "Energy expenditure by cardiac and noncardiac factory workers." In Work and the Heart, (ed) Rosenbaum & Belknap. New York: Hoeber, 1959.

T. V. Parran, "Results of studies at the Work Classification Clinic of the Cleveland Area Heart Society." In Work and the Heart, (ed) Rosenbaum & Belknap. New York: Hoeber, 1959.

H. K. Hellerstein, "Reconditioning and the prevention of heart disease," Modern Med, May 11, 1964.

H. K. Hellerstein, "The influence of active conditioning upon subjects with coronary artery disease: Cardiorespiratory changes during training in 67 patients," Canadian Med Assn J, 96, 1967.

S. H. Salzman, "Serum cholesterol and capacity for physical work of middle-aged sedentary males," Lancet, June 24, 1967.

H. K. Hellerstein, "The influence of active conditioning upon coronary atherosclerosis." In Atherosclerotic Vascular Disease, (ed) Brest & Moyer. New York: Meredith Publishing Co., 1967.

H. K. Hellerstein, "The effects of physical activity. A community program and study among patients and normal coronary prone subjects," Minn Med, 52, 1969.

H. K. Hellerstein, "Exercise therapy in coronary disease, rehabilitation and secondary prevention," VI World Congress of Cardiology, Sept. 6, 1970.

H. K. Hellerstein, "Coronary heart disease—The modern scourge, its recognition and control (Strategy, tactics)," University of Saskatchewan, Saskatoon, Canada, University lecture no. 23, March 1970.

H. K. Hellerstein, "Surviving and thriving with coronary heart disease in 1971. Living, working and loving." Presented at the third public meeting of the Coronary Club, Inc., Cleveland Sheraton Hotel, May 19, 1971.

J. P. Naughton, Exercise Testing and Exercise Training in Coronary Heart Disease. New York: Academic Press, 1973.

H. K. Hellerstein, Exercise & Heart Disease Project: A Collaborative Project." Common Protocol, 1975. The Coordinating Center, The George Washington Medical Center, Washington, DC.

H. K. Hellerstein, "Heart disease and athletics," The Physician & Sportsmedicine, Aug. 1976.

P. S. Fardy, "Benefits of arm exercise in cardiac rehabilitation," The Physician & Sportsmedicine, Oct. 1977.

H. K. Hellerstein, "Acceleration of collaterals due to physical activity—dogma or fact?" Critical Evaluation of Cardiac Rehabilitation, (ed) Kellermann & Denolin. Switzerland: A. G. Basel, 1977.

J. Naughton, "The National Exercise and Heart Disease Project." In Heart Disease and Rehabilitation, (ed) Pollock & Schmidt. Boston: Houghton Mifflin Professional Publishers, 1979.

H. K. Hellerstein, Post Hospital Rehabilitation, (ed) Cohen, Mock, & Ringqvist. New York: John Wiley, 1980.

J. Naughton, "The National Exercise and Heart Disease Project. Interval Report." Sixth International Conference on Cardiac Rehabilitation. Rehabilitation Services Admn., Report no. 4, Cairo, Egypt, 1977.

H. K. Hellerstein, "Exercise prescription for the elderly—normals and cardiac." White House Symposium on Physical Fitness and Sports Medicine. Oct. 11, 1980. Washington Hilton Hotel, Washington, DC.

L. W. Shaw, "Effects of a prescribed supervised exercise program on mortality and cardiovascular morbidity in patients after a myocardial infarction." The National Exercise & Heart Disease Project. Amer J Cardiology, 48, 1981.

H. K. Hellerstein, "Unique insight into problems of cardiovascular rehabilitation which may relate to spaceflight deconditioning and physical fitness." First conference on spaceflight deconditioning and physical fitness. NASA, held in McLean, VA, Jan. 9, 1981.

H. K. Hellerstein, "Exercise testing and prescription." In Rehabilitation of the Coronary Patient, (ed) Wegner & Hellerstein. New York: John Wiley, 1984.

A. Oberman, "Changes in risk factors among participants in long-term exercise rehabilitation program," Adv Cardiology, 31, 1982.

H. K. Hellerstein, "Production, progression, deceleration, and regression of atherosclerosis in humans," Dept. of Med., Case Western Reserve University School of Medicine, Postgraduate course: Medicine, 1984.

CHAPTER 8: TAMERS OF ANGRY BLOOD

Vitamin E: The "Great Hope" Reemerges

M. Scott, "Vitamin E." In Handbook of Lipid Research, vol. 2, (ed) DeLuca. New York: Plenum, 1978.

R. Olson, "Vitamin E and its relation to heart disease," Circulation, 48, 1973.

C. Karpen, "Restoration of prostacyclin/thromboxane balance in the diabetic rat," Diabetes, 31, 1982.

W. Hermann, "The effect of vitamin E on lipoprotein cholesterol distribution," Ann NY Acad Sci, 393, 1982.

R. Gillilan, "Quantitative evaluation of vitamin E in the treatment of angina pectoris," Amer Heart J, 93, 1977.

G. Fitzgerald, "Endogenous prostacyclin and thromboxane biosynthesis during chronic vitamin E therapy in man," Ann NY Acad Sci, 393, 1982.

A. Chan, "Decreased prostacyclin synthesis in vitamin E deficient rabbit aorta," Amer J Clin Nutr, 34, 1981.

J. Barboriak, "Vitamin E supplements and plasma high density lipoprotein cholesterol," Amer J Clin Pathol, 77, 1982.

Vitamin C: The Sour Do-All

E. Ginter, "Ascorbic acid in cholesterol and bile acid metabolism," Ann NY Acad Sci, 258, 1975.

E. Ginter, "Marginal vitamin C deficiency, lipid metabolism and atherogenesis," Adv Lipid Res, 16, 1978.

E. Ginter, "Pretreatment serum cholesterol and response to ascorbic acid," Lancet, 2, 1979.

E. Ginter, "Vitamin C in atherosclerosis," Inter J Vit Nutr Res (suppl.), 19, 1979.

A Bordia, "The effect of vitamin C on blood lipids, fibrinolytic activity and platelet adhesiveness in patients with coronary artery disease," Atherosclerosis, 35, 1980.

H. Heine, "Vitamin C therapy in hyperlipoproteinemia," Int J Vit Nutr Res (suppl.), 19, 1979.

B. Sokoloff, "Effect of ascorbic acid on certain blood fat metabolism factors in animals & man," J Nutr, 91, 1967.

C. Spittle, "Vitamin C and deep vein thrombosis," Lancet, 2, 1973.

Can Folic Acid Help Reverse Heart Disease?

M. R. Malinow, "Prevalence of hyperhomocyst(e)inemia in patients with peripheral arterial occlusive disease," Circulation, 79, 1989.

S. H. Mudd, "Vascular disease and homocysteine metabolism (editorial)," New Eng J Med, 313, 1975.

K. S. McCully, "Vascular pathology of homocysteinemia: Implications for the pathogenesis of arteriosclerosis," Amer J Pathol, 56, 1969.

M. C. Carey, "Homocystinuria: A clinical and pathological study of nine subjects in six families," Amer J Med, 45, 1968.

The Vitamin/Drug Niacin

W. Parsons, "Treatment of hypercholesterolemia by nicotinic acid," Arch Intern Med, 107, 1961.

H. Gurian, "The effect of large doses of nicotinic acid on circulating lipids and carbohydrate tolerance," Amer J Med Sci, 237, 1959.

S. Grundy, "Influence of nicotinic acid on metabolism of cholesterol and triglycerides in man," J Lipid Res, 22, 1981.

B₆: An Artery Protector

J. Rinehart, "Vitamin B$_6$ deficiency in the rhesus monkey with particular reference to the occurrence of atherosclerosis," Amer J Clin Nutr, 4, 1956.

"Is vitamin B$_6$ an antithrombogenic agent?," Lancet, 1, 1981.

"Inhibition of platelet aggregation and clotting by pyridoxal-5 phosphate," Nutr Rev, 40, 1982.

J. Hladovec, "Methionine, pyridoxine and endothelial lesions in rats," Blood Vessels, 17, 1980.

K. McCully, "Homocysteine theory of arteriosclerosis: development and current status," Athero Rev, 11, 1983.

A. Kirksey, "Vitamin B$_6$ nutritional status of a group of female adolescents," Amer J Clin Nutr, 31, 1978.

S. Vir, "Vitamin B$_6$ status of the hospitalized aged," Amer J Clin Nutr, 31, 1978.

The Much-Needed Magnesium

H. Miyagi, "Effect of magnesium on anginal attack induced by hyperventilation in patients with variant angina," Circulation, 79, 1989.

G. Burch, "The importance of magnesium deficiency in cardiovascular disease," Amer Heart J, 94, 1977.

H. Classen, "Magnesium and cardiac necroses," J Intern Acad Prev Med, 6, 1980.

T. Dyckner, "Intracellular potassium after magnesium infusion," Brit Med J, 1, 1978.

T. Dyckner, "Effect of magnesium on blood pressure," Brit Med J, 286, 1983.

P. Elwood, "Myocardial magnesium and ischemic heart disease," Artery, 9, 1981.

L. Iseri, "Magnesium deficiency and cardiac disorders," Amer J Med, 58, 1975.

H. Karppanen, "Epidemiological studies on the relationship between magnesium intake and cardiovascular diseases," Artery, 9, 1981.

R. Masironi, "Epidemiological studies of health effects of water from different sources," Annual Rev Nutr, 1, 1981.

M. Seelig, "Magnesium interrelationships in ischemic heart disease: A review," Amer J Clin Nutr, 27, 1974.

M. Seelig, Magnesium Deficiency in the Pathogenesis of Disease. New York: Plenum Press, 1980.

And, of Course, Aspirin

J. Willis, "Aspirin for heart patients," FDA Drug Bulletin, 15(4), 1985.

M. Abramowicz, "Aspirin to prevent myocardial infarction and death," Med Lett, 28, 1986.

J. M. Ritter, "Therapeutic opportunities in vasoocclusive disease," Circulation, 73, 1986.

J. Hirsh, "Current role of aspirin in CAD," Drug Therapy, 16, 1987.

C. Hennekens, "The Physicians' Health Study: Aspirin and the reduced risk of heart disease," New Eng J Med, Special Report, Jan. 1988.

"International study of infarct survival (ISIS)," Lancet, Aug. 1988.

L. L. Craven, "Acetylsalicyclid acid, possible preventative coronary thrombosis," Annals West Med & Surg, 4, 1950.

F. Bochner, "Is there an optimal dose and formulation of aspirin to prevent arterial thrombo-embolism in man?," Clin Sci, 71, 1986.

J. Hirsh, "The optimal antithrombotic dose of aspirin," Arch Intern Med, 145, 1985.

ACKNOWLEDGMENTS

It is a pleasure to acknowledge my indebtedness to my teachers, mentors, and friends, including Drs. Harold Feil, Harry Goldblatt, Howard T. Karsner, Louis N. Katz, Januk Schlichter, Carl J. Wiggers, Robert Bruce, E. Grey Dimond, Bernard B. Dryer, and the late Thomas Hackett, for their guidance and intellectual stimulation; also to my colleagues and collaborators involved in the activities of the Work Classification Clinic of the Cleveland Area Heart Society, the Cleveland Jewish Community Center-Case Western Reserve Study, and the Staff and Collaborators of the National Exercise and Heart Disease Project. The School of Medicine of Case Western Reserve University and the University Hospitals of Cleveland have enabled my research, clinical practice, and teaching for the past four decades.

My research to which reference is made in this book was supported in part by grants from United States Public Health Services Grant to the Clinical Heart Center of Western Reserve University, HE 06304; Republic Steel Corporation, Grant to the Health Foundation of Greater Cleveland; Rehabilitation Services Administration, Department of Health, Education and Welfare Award Number ORD-RD-P-55917; Rehabilitation Services Administration, Department of Health, Education and Welfare Grant Number 13-P-5738; and National Heart Institute Grant HE 07216.

It is most gratifying to pay tribute to the friendship and grant support of the following, many of whom were also my patients: Mr. and Mrs. Harry Mann, Mr. and Mrs. Harry E. Figgie, Jr., Mr. and Mrs. Donald Krush, Mr. and Mrs. Robert S. Mankin, Mr. and Mrs. Marvin Itts, Mr. and Mrs. Leo Demsey, Mr. and Mrs. David Kangeser, Dr. and Mrs. Benjamin Harlan, Mr. and Mrs. Charles Dussey, Mr. William Luntz, David and Arthur Genshaft, and Francis M. Fine.

It is also a pleasure to praise the contributions to research and professional and public education by the Northern Ohio Affiliate and National American Heart Association and to the American College of Cardiology, and for the opportunity to participate in their local, national, and international activities.

It is also gratifying to express my appreciation for the long-term cooperation and indispensable assistance of Vera M. Husselman, who has served as an administrative assistant through the years of the Case Western Reserve University-Jewish Community Center Study, the National Exercise and Heart Disease Project, and my other academic activities.

Paul Perry and I wish to thank Grace J. Petot, M.S., Assistant Professor of Nutrition, Department of Nutrition and Department of Epidemiology and Biostatistics, School of Medicine Case Western Reserve University, and Suchrita Nelson, M.S., Research Assistant, for their wise counsel, suggestions, and analyses of the dietary diaries, recipes, and menus, employing the Highland View Hospital-Case Western Reserve Nutrient Data Base. We also wish to express our appreciation of the assistance of the publisher and its editorial staff.

Finally, it is a particular delight to express my deepest gratitude to my wife, Mary, and our six children for their love, understanding, and forbearance during the many months and years when my involvement in a multitude of activities often compressed the time we spent together.

—Herman Hellerstein, M.D.

Behind every author is a group of friends, staff, supporters, and even skeptics who make the finished work stronger. Our editor, Bob Bender, has been every one of those things. He has had a great influence on this book, and has proven once again that honest friendship is the best kind. The same can be said for Nat Sobel, our agent. He has been as watchful as a parent through our many projects together.

My wife, Dee, has also had a great influence on this book, both unseen and seen. In addition to making valuable comments on it as a work in progress, she also researched and developed most of the recipes. Her work—along with that of Grace J. Petot, M.S., of the Case Western Reserve University School of Medicine, who provided suggestions and nutritional analysis of the recipes—accounts for food that allows people to make painless but significant changes in their eating habits.

I am deeply indebted to Everette E. Dennis, Executive Director of the Gannett Center for Media Studies at Columbia University. Ev has been a wonderful friend and a great supporter for many years. It was through a Gannett Center fellowship that I was able to study the elements of effective health communication and use most of those techniques in this book.

Special thanks also goes to T George Harris, who as editor-in-chief of *American Health* magazine was always encouraging of my efforts to write about the reversal of heart disease. Gratitude also goes to other staffers at *American Health* magazine, including Joel Gurin, Dana Longstreet, Linda Eger, and Robert Barnett.

My greatest thanks go to Dr. Herman Hellerstein, my coauthor. It is truly his years of experience with the wonders of healing the body and the heart that give this book the human touch.

—Paul Perry

INDEX